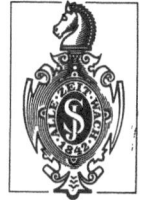

J.-N. Bruneton M. Schneider

Radiology of Lymphomas

With Contributions by
D. Aubanel J.-N. Bruneton E. A. Cabanis
E. Caramella F. Denis J. Drouillard
F. Fauchon J. Frija D. Gardeur M.-T. Iba-Zizen
M.-L. Jablon M. Katz P. Kerboul
M. Laval-Jeantet J.-J. Manzino R. Mashaly
M. Schneider J. Tamraz A. Thyss D. Vanel

Translated by N. Reed Rameau

With a Foreword by J. Tavernier

With 161 Figures and 15 Tables

Springer-Verlag
Berlin Heidelberg GmbH

Editors

Dr. Jean-Noel Bruneton
Prof. Dr. Maurice Schneider
Service de Radiologie, Centre Antoine-Lacassagne
36, Voie Romaine, 06054 Nice Cedex, France

Translator

Nancy Reed Rameau
Centre Antoine-Lacassagne
36, Voie Romaine, 06054 Nice Cedex, France

ISBN 978-3-642-70820-6   ISBN 978-3-642-70818-3 (eBook)
DOI 10.1007/978-3-642-70818-3

Library of Congress Cataloging-in-Publication Data. Main entry under title: Radiology
of lymphomas. Bibliography: p. Includes index. 1. Lymphomas-Diagnosis. 2. Diagnosis,
Radioscopic. I. Bruneton, J.-N. II. Schneider, M. (Maurice), 1933- . III. Aubanel, D.
(Danièle) [DNLM: 1. Lymphoma-radiography. WH 525 R129] RC280.L9R33 1986
616.99′44207572 85-27683

Typesetting, printing, and binding: Appl, Wemding
2121/3140-543210

Foreword

Computerization of the radiological image (digitization, computed tomography), the diagnostic contributions of ultrasonography, and the advent of magnetic resonance imaging all herald a new era in radiology. While this discipline retains its clinical nature, and continues to group together various specialities, the technical "common denominator" plays an increasingly important role, and requires a more global approach to the clinical problem.

Centralization of state-of-the-art equipment in technical imaging centers – strategic points in future hospitals – will allow clinical radiologists to perform all of the examinations required for diagnosis and follow-up with a high degree of reliability, under optimum security, and at the lowest possible cost.

This is the right moment to publish this treatise, as we begin to apply this new approach to radiological studies.

For purposes of clarity, the lymphomatous processes have been dealt with by anatomical location; more important, though, is the discussion of the multiple aspects of diagnosis, with particular emphasis on recent noninvasive modalities (characteristic visceral lesions; analysis and characterization of the anatomical and tissue components of these lesions with the highest possible degree of precision; regional disease extension and anatomical features; information on concomitant regional involvement and distant sites), allowing selection of appropriate therapy and surveillance strategies.

The preponderant roles of ultrasonography and computed tomography, not to mention magnetic resonance imaging, today obviate the need for multiple costly yet unreliable examinations. Indispensable treatment follow-up requires easily repeated noninvasive techniques which furnish sufficient data on the course of disease in lymphomatous sites, while ensuring the maximum degree of comfort for the patient and remaining acceptable costwise.

Jean-Noel Bruneton and Maurice Schneider have succeeded in maintaining this mandatory global approach to the diagnostic, technical, and economic considerations of radiological investigations with the collaboration of radiologists specialized in the various anatomical sites.

Radiology of Lymphomas, the result of considerable experience with the newest techniques and analysis of the most recent findings, is a model for this modern approach to major medical problems. This work attests to the vitality of our discipline, and I sincerely thank the authors.

Jean Tavernier, M.D.
President, University of Bordeaux II

Contents

List of Contributors

Danièle Aubanel
Service de Radiologie, Centre Antoine-Lacassagne
36, Voie Romaine, 06054 Nice Cedex, France

Jean-Noel Bruneton
Service de Radiologie, Centre Antoine-Lacassagne
36, Voie Romaine, 06054 Nice Cedex, France

Emmanuel Alain Cabanis
Service de Radiologie, Hôpital des Quinze-Vingts
28, Rue de Charenton, 75571 Paris Cedex 12, France

Etienne Caramella
Service de Radiologie, Centre Antoine-Lacassagne
36, Voie Romaine, 06054 Nice Cedex, France

François Denis
Service de Radiologie, Centre Antoine-Lacassagne
36, Voie Romaine, 06054 Nice Cedex, France

Jacques Drouillard
Service de Radiologie, Hôpital du Haut-Lévêque
Avenue Magellan, 33600 Pessac, France

François Fauchon
Service de Radiothérapie, Hôpital de la Pitié-Salpêtrière
47–83, Boulevard de l'Hôpital, 75651 Paris Cedex 13, France

Jacques Frija
Service de Radiologie, Hôpital Saint-Louis
2, Place Docteur Alfred-Fournier, 75010 Paris, France

Denis Gardeur
Departement de Scanographie, Clinique de la Roseraie
120, Avenue de la République, 93300 Aubervilliers, France

Marie-Thérèse Iba-Zizen
Service de Radiologie, Hôpital des Quinze-Vingts
28, Rue de Charenton, 75571 Paris Cedex 12, France

Marie-Louise Jablon
Service de Radiologie, Hôpital des Quinze-Vingts
28, Rue de Charenton, 75571 Paris Cedex 12, France

Michel Katz (deceased)
Service de Radiologie, Hôpital Saint-Louis
2, Place Docteur Alfred-Fournier, 75010 Paris, France

Philippe Kerboul
Service de Radiologie, Centre Antoine-Lacassagne
36, Voie Romaine, 06054 Nice Cedex, France

Maurice Laval-Jeantet
Service de Radiologie, Hôpital Saint-Louis
2, Place Docteur Alfred-Fournier, 75010 Paris, France

Jean-Jacques Manzino
Service de Radiologie, Centre Antoine Lacassagne
36, Voie Romaine, 06054 Nice Cedex, France

Ragay Mashaly
Service de Neuro-chirurgie, Hôpital de la Pitié-Salpêtrière
47–83, Boulevard de l'Hôpital, 75651 Paris Cedex 13, France

Maurice Schneider
Service d'Onco-hématologie, Centre Antoine-Lacassagne
36, Voie Romaine, 06054 Nice Cedex, France

Jean Tamraz
Service de Radiologie, Hôpital des Quinze-Vingts
28, Rue de Charenton, 75571 Paris Cedex 12, France

Antoine Thyss
Service d'Onco-hématologie, Centre Antoine-Lacassagne
36, Voie Romaine, 06054 Nice Cedex, France

Daniel Vanel
Service de Radiologie, Institut Gustave-Roussy, Hautes Bruyères
39–53, Rue Camille Desmoulins, 94800 Villejuif, France

1 Classification of Malignant Lymphomas

M. SCHNEIDER AND A. THYSS

Malignant lymphomas, primary tumors of the lymphoid tissues, were first described in 1832 by Thomas Hodgkin. The histological characteristics were later defined by Sternberg and Reed, and Virchow introduced the concept of lymphosarcoma in 1863. Brill and Symmers individualized giant follicular types with a better prognosis, while Oberling, in 1928, isolated the reticulosarcomas (malignant proliferations of reticuloendothelial cells) from lymphosarcomas.

Today, these pathologies are grouped together under the synonymous terms hematosarcoma or malignant lymphoma, which are in turn divided into Hodgkin's disease (HD) and non-Hodgkin's malignant lymphomas (NHL). The average annual incidence of 9.4 per 100000, comparable to that of leukemia, varied only slightly from 1945 to 1970 [466]. HD presents two frequency peaks, one between the ages of 20 and 30 years, the other between the ages of 60 and 70 years [136]. NHL occurs at all ages, its incidence rising progressively after adolescence. As for many other cancers, there is a certain male predominance. Treatment of malignant lymphomas necessitates prior review of the patterns of anatomical distribution and histoprognostic classifications, which vary for each pathology.

1.1 Hodgkin's Disease

HD classically presents as lymphadenopathies, the most frequent sites being the cervical and/or supraclavicular nodes (70% of cases), the axillary nodes (26%), the iliac and inguinal nodes (16%), the mediastinal nodes (62%), the hilar nodes (11%), and the para-aortic nodes [329]. Splenic involvement is less frequent, and even when this organ is enlarged, specific lesions are detected in only one-third of cases [605]. Exploratory laparotomy with splenectomy has permitted spectacular progress in our understanding of the anatomical nature of the disease and its mode of spread. Routine use of this investigative procedure is on the decline, however, owing to the advances obtained with chemotherapy, which lessens the necessity for the accurate localization of lesions [342, 355]. While any of the viscera can be affected by the disease, findings at diagnosis are limited, with lung, liver, bone, pleura, skin, and soft-tissue lesions being noted in only 2%–11% of cases [444, 530].

The physical manifestations include various general symptoms, and in particular fever, night sweats, and weight loss, all of which are of considerable prognostic significance and increase in frequency with disease extension. Biological disorders are also possible, namely concerning the formed elements of the blood, the sedimentation rate, hepatic enzymes, inflammatory proteins, etc. [657]. Impairment of immune responses, and especially impaired cell-mediated immunity, is another well-recognized feature [557].

Positive diagnosis, provided by histology, is always based on the presence of Reed-Sternberg cells [393], the characteristic giant binucleate and nucleolated cells of HD. Jackson and Parker, Lukes and Butler [394], and the 1965 Rye Conference all contributed to the establishment of a histoprognostic classification for HD, divided into four categories depending on the infiltrate associated with the Reed-Sternberg cells. The features of the first type are mature lymphocyte predominance, typical nodal infiltration by histiocytes, eosinophilic granulocytes, and only sparse plasmocytes; lymphocyte predominance accounts for 11%–27% of cases, depending on the author [33, 330, 444, 605]. The second histological type, nodular sclerosis, is characterized by interconnecting bands of collagen within the infiltrate. The Reed-Sternberg cells often have a lacunar appearance. Nodular sclerosing HD is encountered in 31%-71% of cases, depending on the series, and, like lymphocyte predominance, often occurs as localized disease with a favorable prognosis in young adults. This form is highly sensitive to irradiation, but appears less chemosensitive than other types [164]. The remaining two histological types have a less favorable prognosis. Mixed cellularity is characterized by numerous eosinophils, neutrophils, plasmocytes, lymphocytes, and histiocytes. Fibrosis and necrosis are both frequent in this type, which is subdivided into two groups according to whether the infiltrate is nodular or diffuse. Mixed cellularity accounts for 15%-39% of cases. The last histological type, lymphocyte depletion, has the worst histoprognosis. Lymphocytes are scarce, but there are usually numerous Reed-Sternberg cells. Fibrosis is variable. Authors' estimates of this HD form vary from 1% to 19%. Lymphocytic depletion is most often observed in elderly patients presenting with generalized lesions at the time of diagnosis.

Neither the reliability nor the reproducibility of this classification scheme is, however, absolute; in addition to variations that can occur with time, results may also differ from one site to the next when multiple biopsies are obtained. Nodular sclerosis is currently considered a distinct variant of the disease, whereas lymphocyte predominance, mixed cellularity, and lymphocyte depletion are felt to represent more or less related forms [517].

Table 1.1 summarizes the Ann Arbor classification used for topographical clinical staging. The basic premise is that a localized extranodal lesion adjacent to an involved node has the same prognosis as if only the node were involved [444]. In practice, at the time of diagnosis, approximately 60% of locoregional lesions are observed on a single side of the diaphragm [330]. This clinical classification is sometimes completed by a pathological classification based on systematic laparotomy with splenectomy and sampling of multiple subdiaphragmatic nodes plus obtention of liver and bone samples.

The extent of disease spread and the histological type have considerable prognostic value

Table 1.1. Ann Arbor Classification: stages and sub-classification

	Description
Stage I	Involvement of a single lymph node region or of a single extralymphatic organ or site
Stage II	Involvement of two or more lymph node regions on the same side of the diaphragm or localized involvement of an extralymphatic organ or site and of one or more lymph node regions on the same side of the diaphragm. Optionally, the number of node regions involved is indicated by a subscript
Stage III	Involvement of lymph node regions on both sides of the diaphragm. This may or may not be accompanied by localized involvement of an extralymphatic organ or site, involvement of the spleen, or both
Stage III$_1$	Abdominal disease limited to spleen, splenic, celiac, or portal nodes
Stage III$_2$	Abdominal disease involving para-aortic, iliac, or inguinal nodes
Stage IV	Diffuse or disseminated involvement of one or more extralymphatic organs or tissues, with or without associated lymph node involvement. Extralymphatic organs are defined as those other than lymph nodes, spleen, thymus, Waldeyer's ring, appendix and Peyer's patches. Liver and bone marrow involvement always indicate stage IV disease

AB subclassification[a]
Unexplained fever with oral temperature above 38 °C
Night sweats
Unexplained weight loss of 10% or more of body weight in the 6 months before admission

[a] *A* refers to patients without and *B* to patients with these general symptoms

when considered alone, as do such other parameters as sex, age, general signs, anemia, neutrophilia, lymphopenia, erythrocyte sedimentation rate, and diminished immune responses [657]. Various associated signs must also be taken into account and, at present, numerous collaborative studies such as those of the EORTC (European Organization for Research and Treatment of Cancer) emphasize considerable changes in the prognostic value of the different parameters characterizing HD as the result of current therapeutic strategies. Nonetheless, it is fair to state that modern radiotherapy and/or chemotherapy protocols give a 5-year survival rate of 27%–98% depending on the clinical stage, and 17%–90% disease-free survival [330]. Uncontrolled disease involves a succession of relapses with multiple disease sites along with deterioration in general condition, fever, a nephrotic syndrome, cachexia, and infections that are often the immediate cause of death.

1.2 Non-Hodgkin's Malignant Lymphomas

While numerous patients present with nodal involvement at the time of diagnosis, extralymphatic disease sites are also commonly found during initial work-ups. Any of the lymph node groups can be involved, although cervical and supraclavicular sites predominate. The lymphoid formations of the naso-oropharynx are affected in over 10% of cases [94]. Mediastinal lesions are less common than in HD, except in certain histological varieties. By contrast with HD, nodal involvement is often already generalized at the time of diagnosis. After complete initial work-ups, including pedal lymphography, laparotomy, and bone marrow and liver biopsies for 100 patients, Chabner [123] found that less than 15% had disease limited to only local or regional lesions. While neither the liver nor the spleen are usually involved in the early stages of the disease, there have been reports of primary splenic lesions.

Although it is widely recognized that any organ can be involved during the course of NHL it is also known that the first clinical manifestation of the disease may be extralymphatic. Extranodal lesions, seen in 20%–40% of cases depending on the series [532, 544], may be either solitary and/or associated with nodal lesions. Common extranodal sites include the upper respiratory/digestive tracts (nose, sinus, nasopharynx, base of the tongue, mandible, hypopharynx) [94], as well as the salivary, parotid, and thyroid glands. Approximately 10%–20% of the lesions in these sites appear solitary, with no apparent associated nodal involvement.

Orbital lymphomas are not infrequent [345]. Digestive tract lesions, also common, may occur either at the onset of the disease or during the course of its evolution. Gastric and small-bowel disease sites predominate; the colon and rectum are less frequently affected. Jones [317] reported a 16% incidence for gastrointestinal sites in a study of 405 patients.

Other reported primary sites of NHL include the bone, prostate, breast [279], kidney, bladder, ovary, liver, testis, lung, central nervous system and soft tissues [172]. Burkitt's lymphoma, a specific form electively affecting the cheeks and facial bones, warrants separate consideration [87]. As in HD, general symptoms such as asthenia, weight loss, fever, and night sweats are observed in 2%–20% of cases [317, 318]. These symptoms are often directly related to the extent of disease dissemination, and are of unquestionable prognostic value.

From a biological standpoint, the formed elements of the blood are generally normal at the time of diagnosis. Nevertheless, lymphosarcomatous infiltration of the bone marrow is relatively common: 10%–30% of patients present with specific bone marrow infiltration at the time of diagnosis [532], and bilateral bone marrow biopsies should be performed to search for this heterogeneous infiltrate.

During disease progression, numerous extreme variations from normal values may occur in the peripheral blood: leukopenia or leukocytosis, neutropenia, neutrophilia, thrombocytopenia, or anemia, the latter occasionally of autoimmune origin. The passage of lymphosarcomatous cells into the peripheral blood is also fairly common. Other nonspecific serum protein abnormalities are also possible, in particular associated dysglobulinemia.

Bone marrow infiltration by lymphosarcomatous nodules must be distinguished from the leukemic transformations that can take place during the course of the disease, or occasionally right from the start. Both the frequency of such transformations and the morphology of the cells that invade the marrow, then the peripheral blood, depend on the histological type.

The incidence of leukemic transformation, based on large series, is slightly under 10% in adults [532]. The frequency is much higher in children, ranging from 20% to 50% depending on the author [502, 558].

By contrast with HD, the prognosis of NHL is less correlated with the extent of disease. Clinical staging using the Ann Arbor classification is of less formal value, since disseminated nodal and/or visceral lesions can be found in the majority of patients if investigations are pursued far enough and with enough attention to detail. Moreover, certain forms, despite widespread lesions, progress very slowly, while other forms, despite initially limited lesions, have extremely poor prognoses [533].

The prognosis actually depends above all on the histological form of the disease. Unfortunately, although numerous histological schemes have been proposed for the classification of NHL, none of them has proven entirely satisfactory. In most cases, the cells in which the disease originates belong to the lymphocytic line, although their degree of differentiation varies from patient to patient. The cell population may be monomorphous or mixed, and infiltration may occur either diffusely or in a nodular (follicular) manner roughly resembling a lymphoid follicle. The first classifications divided NHL into three groups: lymphocytic lymphosarcoma, reticulum cell sarcoma, and giant follicular lymphosarcoma. In 1956, Rappaport devised a scheme which he continued to modify until 1966 [515] (Table 1.2). This classification is based on cell morphology and the architecture of the infiltrate (nodular or diffuse). One of its consequences was to eliminate Brill-Symmers disease as a specific entity, since this pathology corresponds to the nodular or follicular forms of NHL. Rappaport's classification continues to be the most commonly used worldwide, owing to its simplicity, reproducibility, and prognostic value. In particular, it reflects the more favorable outlook for nodular and well-differentiated lymphocytic forms.

The term "histiocyte," used by Rappaport, evokes the morphology of certain cells viewed

by light microscopy. Recent progress in immunology, though, has demonstrated that in the majority of cases the large cells having the appearance of histiocytes are actually transformed lymphocytes, and that true reticulum cell sarcomas exist only in very small numbers.

New immunological techniques now allow determination of the degree of lymphoid cell maturity and differentiation. Classification as T, B, or null cells is based on the use of markers such as membrane immunoglobulins, receptors for sheep erythrocytes or intracellular elements, and, more recently, highly specific monoclonal antibodies, which accurately distinguish cell surface membrane antigens [206].

Schematically, lymph nodes comprise the following three zones [649]:

1. Primary and secondary lymphoid follicles of the cortical areas, composed of B-lymphocytes.
2. The marginal and interfollicular zones, in which the lymphocytes may be activated and transformed into immunoblasts (large nucleolated cells with a basophilic cytoplasm) and plasmocytes.
3. The paracortical zones composed of T-lymphocytes.

Immunological criteria can also be employed to characterize the cells involved in NHL. The nodular forms of the Rappaport classification are generally type B [303]. Diffuse lymphomas include a wide variety of cell types. Diffuse poorly and well-differentiated lymphocytic lymphomas are generally type B. Mixed histiocytic and undifferentiated types involve B cells in 50%-60% of cases, T cells in 15%, and null cells in 15%-25% [206].

Based on immunological characterization, Lukes and Collins [395] suggested that NHL corresponds to abnormalities in lymphocyte transformation in response to antigenic stimuli (Table 1.3). The new classification they drew up as a result is widely used in the United States. The most unfavorable prognoses are associated with the small noncleaved, large noncleaved, T-convoluted lymphocytic, B and T immunoblastic sarcoma, and unclassified cell types [395].

The Kiel classification [230, 371], which introduced the terms centrocyte/centroblast for

Table 1.2. NHL: Rappaport classification (1966)

Lymphocytic, well differentiated
Lymphocytic, poorly differentiated
Mixed lymphocytic and histiocytic
Histiocytic
Undifferentiated

Nodular or diffuse

Table 1.3. Lukes and Collins classification of NHL

T-malignant lymphomas	Small lymphocytic
	Convoluted lymphocytic
	Sezary's syndrome – mycosis fungoides
	Immunoblastic sarcoma
B-malignant lymphomas	Small lymphocytic (CLL)
	Plasmacytoid lymphocytic
	Follicular center cell:
	– Small cleaved
	– Large cleaved
	– Small noncleaved
	– Large noncleaved
	Immunoblastic sarcoma
Histiocytic	
Unclassified	

CLL, chronic lymphocytic leukemia

Table 1.4. Kiel classification of NHL

Low-grade malignant lymphomas	Lymphocytic
	Lymphoplasmacytic/cytoid (immunocytoma)
	Centrocytic
	Centrocytic/centroblastic:
	– Follicular
	– Follicular ± diffuse
	– Diffuse
	Unclassified
High-grade malignant lymphomas	Centroblastic
	Lymphoblastic
	– Burkitt's type
	– Convoluted cell type
	– Unclassified
	Immunoblastic
	Unclassified
Composite lymphoma	

NHL arising in lymphoid follicles, emphasizes cell morphology rather than the nodular or diffuse pattern of infiltration. A distinction is made between the prognoses for low-grade and high-grade lymphomas (Table 1.4). Low-grade malignant lymphomas consist of "cytes," but may also contain a certain number of "blasts," whereas high-grade malignant lymphomas contain only "blasts."

The WHO classification [424], also based on cell morphology (Table 1.5) and the topographic aspects of proliferation, likewise distinguishes a certain number of forms with a poor outlook (high-grade): diffuse immunoblastic, diffuse Burkitt's tumor, and diffuse lymphoblastic.

Additional classifications have been suggested by Bennett et al. [42], Diebold [167], and Dorfman [169].

This multiplicity of classifications considerably complicates matters for pathologists and clinicians alike. At present, comparison of therapeutic trials can prove difficult, since the patient populations may have been established using different criteria. Another problem with these classifications is the fact that they deal only partially with NHL in children; for example, childhood stage I and II disease usually has a more favorable prognosis. Likewise, nodular forms and well differentiated lymphocytic lymphosarcomas are exceptional in children [90]. Lymphoblastic lymphosarcomas with me-

Table 1.5. WHO classification of NHL

Nodular lymphosarcoma, prolymphocytic
Nodular lymphosarcoma, prolymphocytic-lymphoblastic
Diffuse lymphosarcoma, lymphocytic
Diffuse lymphosarcoma, lymphoplasmacytic
Diffuse lymphosarcoma, prolymphocytic
Diffuse lymphosarcoma, prolymphocytic-lymphoblastic
Diffuse lymphosarcoma, lymphoblastic
Diffuse lymphosarcoma, immunoblastic
Diffuse lymphosarcoma, Burkitt's tumor
Mycosis fungoides
Plasmacytoma
Reticulosarcoma
Malignant lymphoma, unclassified
Composite lymphoma

diastinal infiltration account for one-third of cases affecting children; on an immunological level, the T cells involved frequently undergo leukemic transformation, and the general prognosis is still poor despite aggressive chemotherapy [206]. NHL in children often originates from B-lymphocytes, the majority being classified as Burkitt's type with prominent abdominal symptomatology.

In response to the problems encountered with disease classification, a major study organized by the National Cancer Institute involving specialists from numerous institutions compared the six main classifications in connection with the complete records of 1175 patients. The result of this study was the "Working Formulation for Clinical Usage" [608], which uses purely morphologic criteria to divide NHL into ten major types grouped in three prognostic grades (Table 1.6). This working formulation is proposed not as a new classification scheme, but rather as a means of "translating" data from one of the existing systems to another, thus facilitating clinical comparison of case reports and clinical trials.

The evolutionary course of NHL is nearly impossible to summarize in an overall manner. The median survival for the histologically favorable forms in Rappaport's classification, i.e., well-differentiated lymphocytic forms close to chronic lymphoid leukemia and Waldenström's disease, varies from 3 to 12 years [191]. Depending on the extent of disease, radiotherapy and/or single- or multi-agent chemotherapy is indicated, the latter treatments usually being only slightly aggressive. The prognosis for nodular forms is also good, with 70% survival at 5 years, but the survival curves show no plateaus and no cures have yet been found [7]. The utility of aggressive treatments for nodular forms remains the subject of controversy, even though certain studies emphasize the benefits of obtaining a remission. The validity of treatment for asymptomatic patients is also questioned by certain authors, owing to the indolent course of many lymphomas [506]. Results for histologically unfavorable forms are highly disparate. Exclusive radiotherapy has occasionally produced up to 78% disease-free survival at 5 years for truly localized stages [48]. Today, however, use of chemotherapy/radiotherapy combinations is almost universal [57], with chemotherapy occasionally being used alone [92] and providing 90% disease-free survival at 5 years.

Table 1.6. Working formulation for clinical usage in the classification of NHL

Low grade	Malignant lymphoma, small lymphocytic
	Malignant lymphoma, follicular, predominantly small cleaved cell
	Malignant lymphoma, follicular, mixed, small cleaved and large cell
Intermediate grade	Malignant lymphoma, follicular, predominantly large cell
	Malignant lymphoma, diffuse, small cleaved cell
	Malignant lymphoma, diffuse, mixed, small and large cell
	Malignant lymphoma, diffuse, large cell
High grade	Malignant lymphoma, large cell, immunoblastic
	Malignant lymphoma, lymphoblastic
	Malignant lymphoma, small non-cleaved cell
Miscellaneous	Composite
	Mycosis fungoides
	Histiocytic
	Extramedullary plasmacytoma
	Unclassifiable
	Other

Chemotherapy is the main treatment for disseminated forms; the major associations include doxorubicin hydrochloride (Adriamycin), cyclophosphamide, vincristine sulfate, methotrexate, and prednisone. Radiotherapy is used more for adjuvant purposes. Synthesis of recent studies allows us to reasonably expect 40% relapse-free survival at 10 years and the establishment of a cure plateau in the near future [505].

2 Lymphomas of the Central Nervous System

D. GARDEUR, R. MASHALY, AND F. FAUCHON

2.1 Intracranial Lymphomas

Computed tomography (CT) has transformed the radiological exploration of cerebral lymphomas. In addition to detecting tumors, which are often primary, CT demonstrates such lymphoma-related complications as ischemia, hemorrhage, infections, and therapy-related complications (Table 2.1).

2.1.1 Tumoral Infiltration

The frequency of intracranial malignant lymphomas varies with the histological type: the incidence is very high for Burkitt's lymphoma, relatively high for certain non-Hodgkin's lymphomas (NHL; diffuse histiocytic, diffuse poorly differentiated), but extremely low for Hodgkin's disease (HD). Primary cerebral lymphomas are a separate entity, and are caused by various histological types.

2.1.1.1 Lymphomatous Meningitis

Infiltration of the leptomeningeal spaces [170, 221, 264] occurs during the course of 4%–7% of malignant lymphomas; it is more common in NHL than in HD (approximately 2% of cases). The highest frequencies of leptomeningeal disease sites (30%–50%) are seen in diffuse histiocytic, diffuse poorly differentiated, or undifferentiated NHL, in primary cerebral lymphomas, and especially in Burkitt's lymphoma.

The CT appearance generally remains normal in cases of lymphomatous meningitis. Enhancements of abnormal tissue by iodinated contrast material are visible only in instances of extensive dural infiltration or disruption of the pial-glial barrier with intracerebral tumoral infiltration. Secondary hydrocephalus with cisternal stenosis is rare. Diagnosis of lymphomatous leptomeningeal infiltration relies on clinical findings and cytologic analysis of lumbar punctures.

Table 2.1. Clinical Manifestations of the neurological complications of lymphomas

Type of complication	Clinical signs	Lumbar puncture	Other examinations
Tumoral infiltration			

Lymphomatous meningitis	Cranial nerve involvement:
	  – Oculomotor nerves
	  – Optic nerve
	Nerve root involvement:
	  – Sciatic nerve
	Discrete meningeal syndrome
		Elevation of proteins
		  in the CSF
		Specific cells
		Elevation of carcinoembryonic antigen
		  in the CSF	

Metastatic epiduritis	Spinal involvement (often dorsal)		
Peripheral neuropathy	Onset often subacute or acute Polyneuritis	Normal	Neuromuscular biopsy: specific infiltration
Intracerebral sites	Multifocal symptoms: 30% Sensory and motor deficit, aplasia } 50% Frontal syndrome Intracranial hypertension, epilepsy, posterior fossa signs (dysarthria, ataxia): 20%	Not recommended	EEG: slow wave areas or signs of diffuse encephalopathy

Table 2.1 *(continued)*

Type of complication	Clinical signs	Lumbar puncture	Other examinations
Vascular complications			
Arterial thrombosis	Acute development of symptoms corresponding to arterial ischemia	Normal except in cases of hemorrhagic cerebral infarcts	
Venous thrombosis	Superior longitudinal sinus: – Pure intracranial hypertension – Ischemia in a nonarterial territory Seizures	Elevation in CSF pressure	
Intracranial hemorrhage	Seizures Deficit with meningeal signs and impaired vigilance	Not recommended	
Bacterial infections			
Purulent meningitis	Severe meningeal syndrome Fever, stiffness, headache, vomiting	Decrease in glycorrhachia Cellular elements: 1000–2000 altered polynuclear cells/mm^3 Protein: 1–5 g/l Culture: germs detected	
Brain abscess	Febrile state Focal signs of rapid onset Epilepsy Intracranial hypertension	Not recommended	
Tuberculosis			
Tuberculous meningitis	Deterioration in general condition Meningeal signs	Glycorrhachia <3 mmol/l Protein: up to 1 g/l Cellular elements: 10–350 mononuclear and polymorphous cells/mm^3 Culture on Löwenstein-Jensen medium	
Tuberculoma	Deterioration in general condition Focal signs: frontal, parietal or occipital Brain stem signs Seizures	Often normal	
Mycoses			
Meningitis caused by cryptococcosis	Deterioration in general condition: fever, stiffness	Elevation of proteins in the CSF Cellular elements: 10–100 lymphocytes/mm^3 Culture on Sabouraud's agar	
Candidiasis	Encephalitis stage: diffuse signs Abscess stage: focal signs	Specific immunofluorescence	Serologic immunodiffusion and immunofluorescence

Table 2.1 *(continued)*

Type of complication	Clinical signs	Lumbar puncture	Other examinations
Viral infections			
Herpetic encephalitis	Febrile condition Temporal focal signs with impaired vigilance Generalized or temporal epilepsy	Cellular reaction: <50 elements/mm^3 (lymphocytes, polynuclear cells) Elevation of proteins in the CSF	EEG: periodic activity on the 3rd–5th days, disappearing around the 15th day
Progressive multifocal leukoencephalopathy	Unifocal signs: 12% Diffuse signs: character disorder progressing to dementia: 80% Course: 3–6 months	Normal or elevation of proteins in the CSF	Diffuse slow signs, exceeding the clinical localizing signs
Subacute sclerosing panencephalitis	Decrease in mental efficiency Epilepsy Myoclonia Pyramidal and extrapyramidal signs	Elevation of gamma globulins Elevation of antimeasles antibodies	EEG: periodic complexes, diphasic slow waves
Granulomatous angiitis	Diffuse signs of mental deterioration: 70% Focal signs: 30% Intracranial hypertension: rare Rare medullary signs: 2/29	Elevation of proteins in the CSF: 70% Cellular reaction (lymphocyte: 65%)	
Parasitosis			
Cerebral toxoplasmosis	Meningoencephalitis: 50% with diffuse signs and impaired consciousness Cerebral mass: 50% with focal signs	Elevation of proteins in the CSF in 60% of cases Cellular reaction: between 6 and 60 lymphocytes/mm^3 IgG, IgM tests	Specific serologic test; must be repeated when negative
Iatrogenic complications			
Radiation-induced myelopathy	Regressive forms: paresthesia Stabilized forms: pyramidal and posterior spinal cord disorders Progressive forms: paraparesis with motor and sensory disorders	Normal	
Necrotizing leukoencephalopathy	Reversible forms: mental confusion, improvement with corticosteroids Stable forms: sequelae of mental deterioration Fatal progressive forms (rare): coma and death within 4 months	Elevation in basic proteins	
Drug toxicity	Vincristine: peripheral neuropathy L-asparaginase: reversible somnolence and mental confusion Procarbazine hydrochloride: mental confusion Cyclophosphamide: inappropriate antidiuretic hormone secretion	Normal Normal Normal	EEG: signs of diffuse encephalopathy

2.1.1.2 Dural Infiltration

Dural infiltration (Figs. 2.1 and 2.2 [310, 447]) is more common in HD (up to 7% of cases) than in NHL. Primary dural lymphomas are rare. The majority of dural lesions are contiguous to an osseous lesion of the base of the skull or ver-

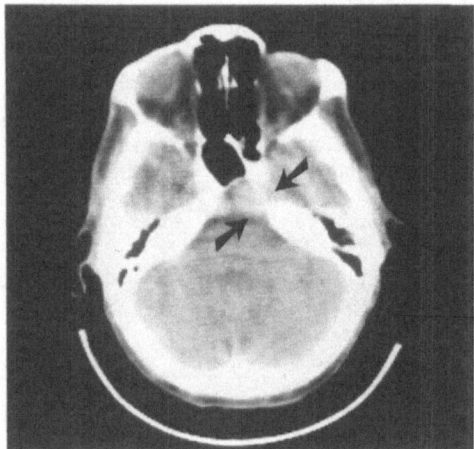

Fig. 2.1. Dural involvement secondary to a lymphomatous bone lesion: lysis of the clivus and abnormal enhancement of the posterior left cavernous sinus and the retroclival region *(arrows)*

tex; involvement of the falx is exceptional. CT demonstrates dural lymphomatous sites as discretely hyperdense juxta-osseous masses; following injection of iodinated contrast material, these lesions enhance in an intense, homogeneous manner. Dural masses are usually rather well demarcated from the adjacent cerebral parenchyma, and are occasionally surrounded by cerebral edema secondary to venous thrombosis or secondary cerebral infiltration. Small dural infiltrations near the base of the skull or the superior convexity are sometimes visible only on coronal CT scans.

2.1.1.3 Intracerebral Sites

Intracerebral sites [10, 64, 170, 188, 224, 264, 236, 339, 350, 447, 481, 483, 513, 584, 591, 601, 610, 614, 654] (Figs. 2.3–2.5) of HD are exceptional (less than 1% of cases); the incidence is higher for NHL. Cerebral lymphomas are generally primary lesions, and account for approximately 1% of adult brain tumors (literature figures range from 0,2% to 2%). This type of tumor is referred to by a multitude of denominations in the literature: primary cerebral reticulum cell sarcoma, microglioma, perithelial sarcoma, histiocytic lymphoma, etc. Cerebral tu-

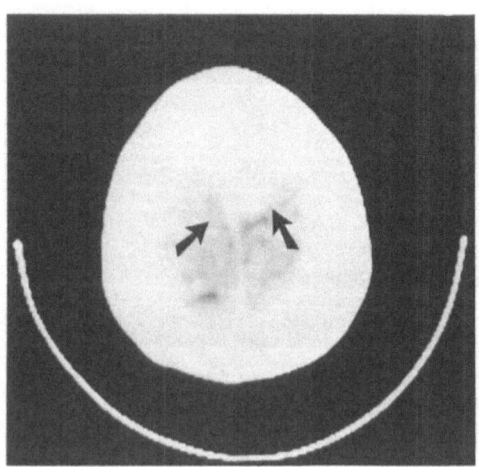

Fig. 2.2. Dural site of lymphoma *(arrows)*

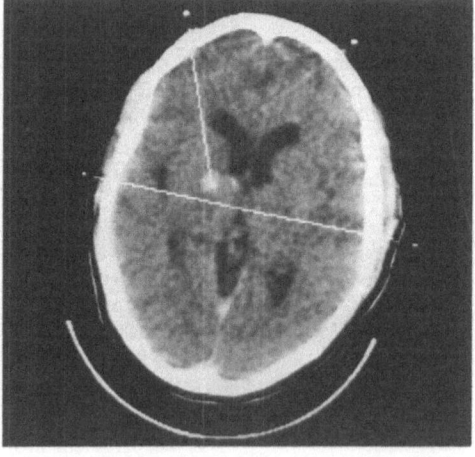

Fig. 2.3. Cerebral lymphomatous site: following contrast medium injection, CT demonstrated abnormal hyperdense lesions in the right foramen of Monro, the head of the left caudate nucleus, and within the brain stem. Stereotaxic brain biopsy was performed following centering by CT. *White lines,* scales for therapy purposes

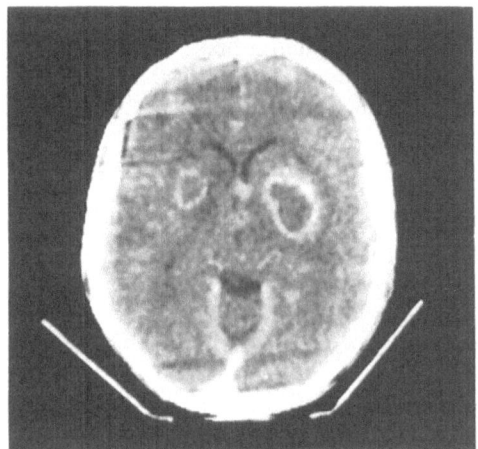

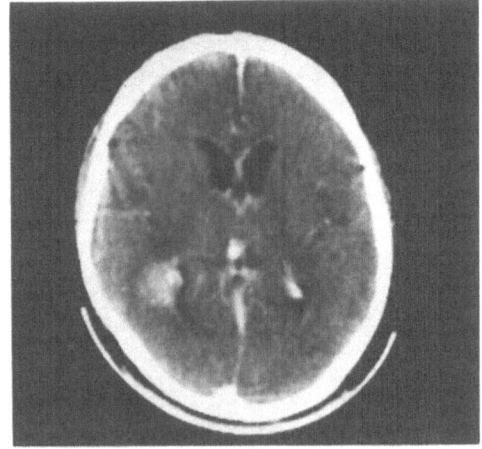

Fig. 2.4. Onset of right hemiplegia and aphasia in a case of HD in remission for 7 years: postcontrast CT revealed multiple hyperdense intracerebral masses, the largest located in the left lentiform nucleus

Fig. 2.5. Sudden onset of character disorder in a patient with treated NHL: CT evidenced a mass near the left ventricular trigone, with enhancement of the ventricular walls indicating subependymal spread of tumor

mors are especially common in immunodeficient individuals (particularly cardiac and renal transplant recipients). Primary and secondary cerebral lymphomas show a variety of CT appearances.

Intracerebral Masses. The most frequent manifestation, intracerebral masses may be solitary or multiple; their anatomical distribution (Table 2.2) and CT features (Table 2.3) are characteristic. Intracerebral masses are often located around the lateral ventricles (central gray nuclei, corpus callosum, septum pellucidum), although other sites are also suggestive: the vermis cerebelli, frontal white matter, hypothalamus, and brain stem. Subcortical masses and lesions deep within the white matter are less frequent. These tumoral masses are usually spontaneously isodense or moderately hyperdense. Following the injection of contrast medium, enhancement is intense and usually homogeneous. Tumor nodules are well demarcated from the uninvolved cerebral parenchyma; their contours are sometimes irregular and slightly blurred. Intracerebral masses are often surrounded by more or less extensive edema, although the latter is usually minimal in comparison to the size of the tumor. Certain deep cerebral lymphomas do not elicit any edematous reaction. Solitary lymphomatous masses

Table 2.2. Anatomical distribution of 79 cases of cerebral lymphoma (primary and secondary) diagnosed by CT[a]

Location	Number
Occipital, parietal and/or temporal	14
Central gray nuclei, thalamus	23
Corpus callosum, septum pellucidum	16
Subependymal, periventricular	14
Hypothalamus	7
Brain stem	3
Cerebellum	8
Multiple sites	32

[a] Literature review plus personal observations

Table 2.3. CT appearance of cerebral lymphomas (primary and secondary)[a]

1. Spontaneous densities	hypodense	16%
	isodense	16.5%
	hyperdense	42%
	mixed	25.5%
2. Contrast enhancement		95%
3. Central hypodense areas following injection of iodinated contrast material		22%
4. Perilesional edema		76%

[a] Literature review plus personal observations

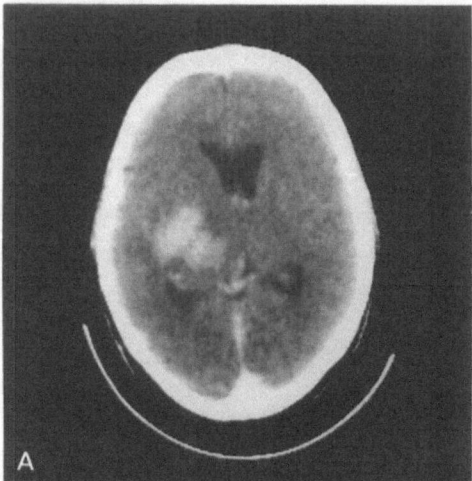

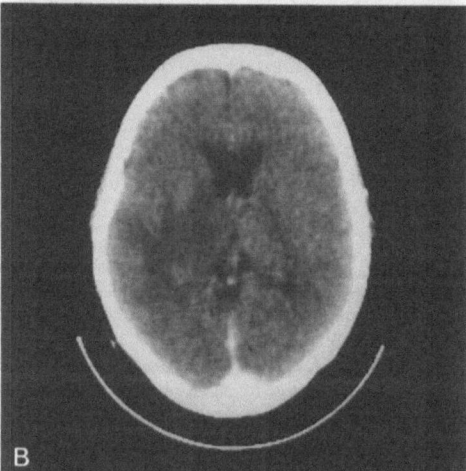

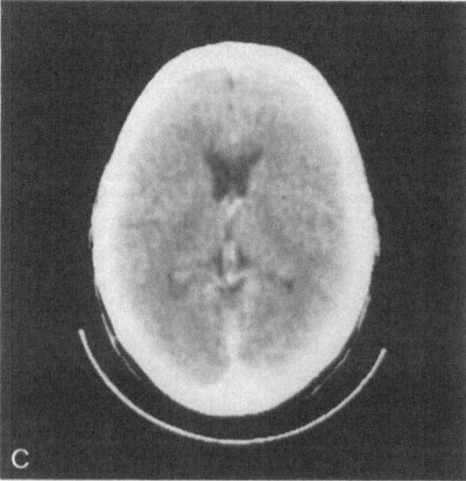

are slightly more frequent than multiple lesions. Bilateral mirror-image tumoral involvement of the central gray nuclei is a suggestive but inconstant finding.

Infiltrative Forms. The following signs combine in infiltrative forms, which are less common: large hypodense cerebral patches with no identifiable enhancement, and diffuse subependymal enhancement lining the ventricular walls and/or diffuse gyriform cortical enhancement of leptomeningeal infiltrations. Cerebral arteriography generally reveals only indirect signs (mass effect on vessels); a rather homogeneous tumor blush is occasionally visible, but neovascularity and arteriovenous fistulas are rare.

The differential diagnosis of primary cerebral lymphomas can be difficult. Possible diagnoses for multiple lesions include metastases of visceral tumors and unrecognized melanomas; metastases, however, are rarely periventricular, and usually cause much more extensive cerebral edema than do lymphomas. Less frequent differential diagnoses include multiple sclerosis and neurosarcoidosis. Solitary lesions may suggest glioblastoma, but the latter pathology often exhibits low-density centers. While the differential diagnosis for certain deep meningiomas can prove difficult, since their CT appearances are similar to those of lymphomas, meningeal lesions are more frankly intraventricular. In cases of acquired immune deficiency syndrome (AIDS), brain biopsy is required to distinguish cerebral toxoplasmosis from lymphoma. Tumors of the posterior cranial fossa can be confused with medulloblastoma, meningioma, or even neurinoma. Pituitary adenoma and hypothalamic glioma can be enter-

◁ **Fig. 2.6 A–C.** Progressive left hemiplegia in an NHL patient. **A** CT demonstrated a large enhancing right inferior lenticular-thalamic mass. **B** The first surveillance CT scan after radiotherapy revealed disappearance of the enhancement, but persistence of a deep hypodense area and compression of the right ventricular trigone. **C** After 40 Gy, the second surveillance CT study showed disappearance of the intracerebral lymphomatous involvement

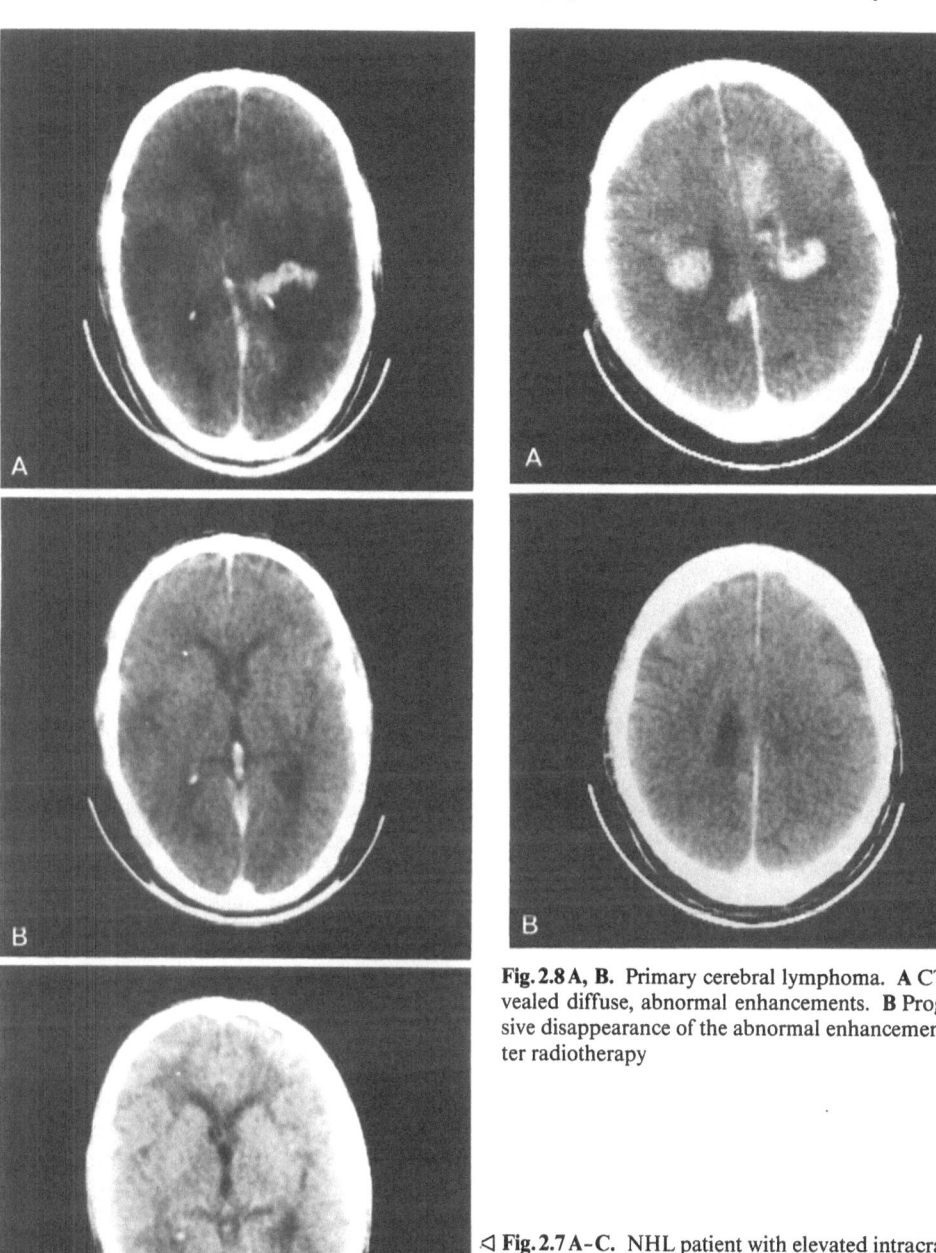

Fig. 2.8 A, B. Primary cerebral lymphoma. **A** CT revealed diffuse, abnormal enhancements. **B** Progressive disappearance of the abnormal enhancement after radiotherapy

◁ **Fig. 2.7 A–C.** NHL patient with elevated intracranial pressure and right hemiparesis. **A** CT demonstrated a cerebral mass near the ventricular trigone surrounded by extensive edema. **B** One month after radiotherapy, the cerebral mass had disappeared. **C** Two years later, there was no tumoral recurrence, but diffuse hypodense white matter areas corresponded to radiation-induced leukoencephalopathy

tained as possible diagnoses for solitary suprasellar lesions. Possible diagnoses for infiltrating forms exhibiting diffuse subependymal enhancement include medulloblastoma, pinealoma, and ependymoma. Since cerebral lymphomas are usually extremely radiosensitive, accurate diagnosis is vital. A brain biopsy is warranted whenever the diagnosis is equivocal, especially for deep lesions. CT is highly useful for monitoring tumor response to radiotherapy, which can induce spectacular tumor regressions (Figs. 2.6–2.8). Specific chemotherapy and corticosteroid treatments can also bring about regression of intracerebral masses.

2.1.2 Iatrogenic Lesions

2.1.2.1 Subacute Necrotizing Leukoencephalopathy

Subacute necrotizing encephalopathy (SNL) [220, 221, 350], a white matter disease, may occur secondary to associations of cerebral radiotherapy and intrathecal methotrexate. Radiotherapy appears to promote intracerebral methotrexate diffusion by transiently opening the blood-brain barrier. The current rise in the incidence of SNL is the result of both longer patient survival and improved lesion detection thanks to CT. CT demonstrates SNL as diffuse hypodense areas in the white matter; both cerebral hemispheres are involved more or less symmetrically, and lesions predominate in the periventricular region, the semioval center, and the frontal white matter. In acute stages, the hypodense areas in the white matter are essentially edematous, and can cause a mass effect on the ventricular system. Lesions are occasionally reversible at this stage.

In a later stage, the hypodense areas become more marked and more focal, reflecting white matter demyelination and necrosis; in severe cases, they may no longer be directly visible. Dilatation of the lateral ventricles may now appear, and be associated with various degrees of sulcal-cisternal widening. Injection of contrast material generally does not reveal any modifications in density, although ringlike enhancement simulating an abscess or a brain tumor has been reported in acute inflammatory and edematous forms. Intracerebral calcification

can occur in chronic stages. Located in areas of white matter necrosis, calcification reflects the associated mineralizing microangiopathy. Calcification is usually a diffuse process seen in subcortical sites, although both the cortex and central gray nuclei can also be affected.

2.1.2.2 Other Leukoencephalopathies

Diffuse hypodense areas in the white matter suggestive of diffuse leukoencephalopathies can be observed following exclusive radiotherapy, without any associated methotrexate administration. Such findings generally correspond to occasionally reversible edematous cerebral lesions, although diffuse demyelination with ventricular dilatation is also possible. True radionecrosis and intracerebral pseudotumors are exceptional, since the radiation doses given for cerebral lymphomas are not very high.

2.1.2.3 Cerebral Atrophy

Sulcal-cisternal widening with more or less extensive ventricular dilatation is frequent during the course of intracranial lymphomas. Such phenomena, which suggest cerebral atrophy [62, 220, 221] prior to diagnosis, have various etiologies:

Cerebral radiotherapy

Tumoral involution and a decrease in ventricular volume

Intrathecal or intravenous chemotherapy (Fig. 2.9)

Corticosteroid therapy (but sulcal widening is reversible on withdrawal of steroids)

Leptomeningeal lymphomatous infiltration that can mimic cerebral atrophy

External hydrocephalus secondary to tumoral meningitis of the convexity or to venous thrombosis

Multiple cerebral arterial infarcts

Paraneoplastic cerebral atrophy

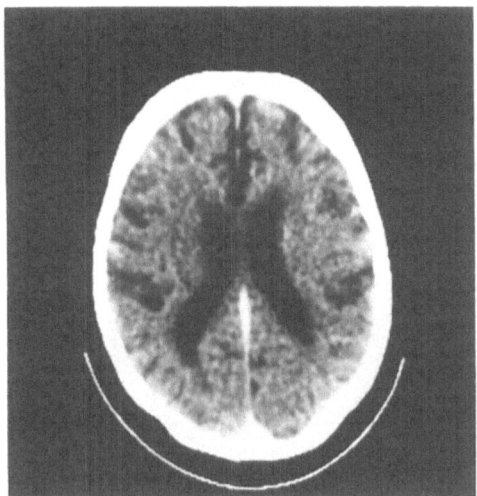

Fig. 2.9. NHL treated by chemotherapy: corticosubcortical cerebral atrophy

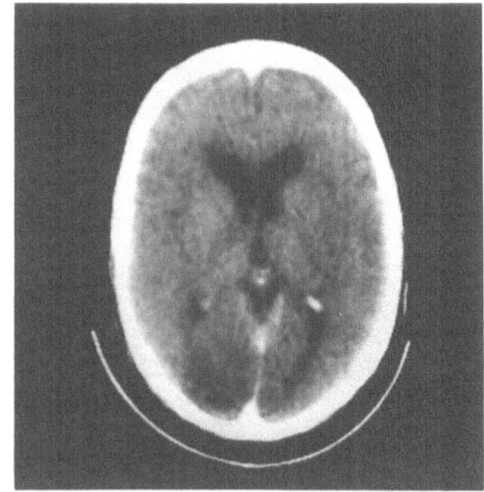

Fig. 2.10. NHL treated by chemotherapy: multiple right capsulothalamic and occipital ischemic cerebral lesions

2.1.3 Intracranial Vascular Lesions

2.1.3.1 Arterial Thrombosis

Occlusion of cerebral arteries [356] is rare but not exceptional in lymphomas. Provided the occluded artery is sufficiently proximal, CT can evidence signs of cerebral ischemia (hypodense areas and/or gyriform enhancement; Figs. 2.10 and 2.11). Cerebral ischemia is quite often hemorrhagic, because of associated coagulation disorders; it can occur secondary to radiation angiitis, namely after cervical irradiation. Digital angiography is indicated in such cases, to determine the condition of the cervical carotid arteries. Occlusion of more distal arteries, encountered especially in cases of granulomatous angiitis with herpes zoster infection, causes diffuse, nonfocal cerebral lesions, which are initially edematous but subsequently become atrophic. Carotid arteriography can sometimes demonstrate segmental arterial narrowing.

2.1.3.2 Venous Thrombosis

Venous thrombosis occurs secondary to tumoral infiltration of the sinuses of the dura mater or to abnormal intravascular coagulation. Thrombosis of the superior longitudinal sinus

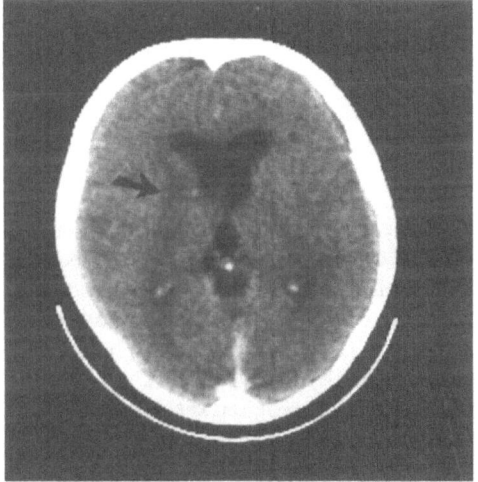

Fig. 2.11. Sudden onset of left hemiplegia in a patient with NHL: right internal capsular hypodensity of ischemic origin *(arrow)*

(Fig. 12 B), the most frequent site, causes intracranial hypertension and/or venous infarcts which are usually hemorrhagic (Fig. 12 A). Diagnosis can be made by postcontrast CT scans, which demonstrate a hypodense triangular formation in the superior longitudinal sinus, but the preferred diagnostic technique at present is digital angiography. Focal cortical venous thrombosis is difficult to differentiate from pri-

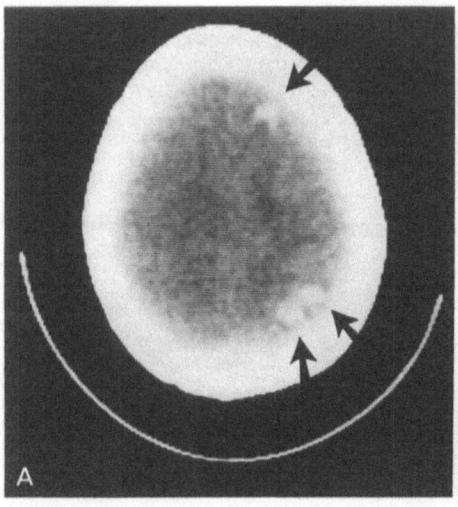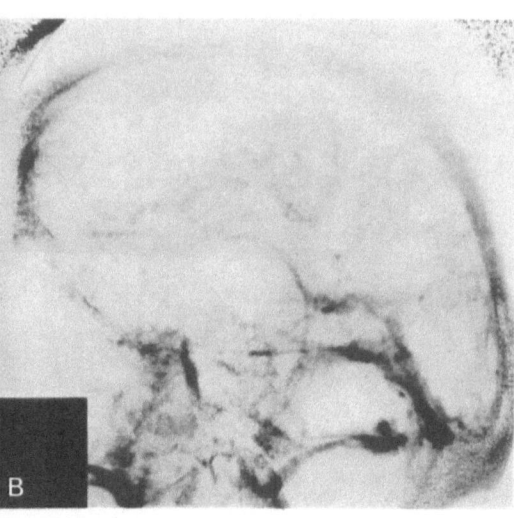

Fig. 2.12 A, B. Sudden onset of repeated seizures. A CT demonstrated hyperdense cortical lesions *(arrows)* suggestive of hemorrhagic cerebral infarcts.

B Digital angiography revealed complete thrombosis of the superior longitudinal sinus (lateral view)

mary intracerebral hemorrhage and hemorrhagic ischemia of arterial origin.

2.1.3.3 Intracranial Hemorrhage

The causes of intracranial hemorrhage include hemorrhagic ischemia secondary to arterial or venous occlusion, intratumoral hemorrhage, and intracerebral hemorrhage secondary to blood dyscrasias or septic vasculopathies. CT can easily diagnose intracranial hemorrhage (spontaneous hyperdense areas), provided that the accident is recent and that the hemoglobin concentration is sufficiently high.

2.1.4 Infectious Complications

Intracranial infections [220] are quite common complications of malignant lymphomas. In addition to infections by common germs, atypical infections often develop in immunocompromised patients, owing to opportunistic organisms that are normally nonpathogenic or of low pathogenicity.

2.1.4.1 Bacterial Infections

Meningitis caused by *Listeria* or gram-negative bacilli predominates, but pyogenic brain abscesses can also develop.

Purulent Meningitis. The CT appearance is often normal when purulent meningitis is investigated during the early stages or after rapid, successful treatment. Less frequent CT abnormalities include widening of the subarachnoid spaces, superficial gyriform enhancement, ventricular dilatation, and cerebral hypodense areas. The only justification for CT investigation of acute purulent meningitis is the search for possible complications. Likewise, once a certain interval has elapsed after the initial episode, CT is occasionally indicated to detect possible extracerebral collections, brain abscess, or hydrocephalus.

Brain Abscesses. The CT appearance of brain abscesses depends on the stage of development. Presuppurative encephalitis is demonstrated as heterogeneous, poorly circumscribed hypodense cerebral areas showing heterogeneous enhancement. Once purulent collections have formed, a ring-shaped enhancement pattern is usually visible; the usually thin, uniform ring surrounds a distinct low-density center, and is itself surrounded by an edematous hypo-dense area. Purulent collections in patients who are immunosuppressed and/or on corti-costeroid therapy do not always show ring en-hancement on CT scans; heterogeneous lesions in these patients can correspond to an encapsu-lated abscess [189, 201]. Neither carotid arteri-ography nor radionuclide brain scans provide any supplemental information for the diagno-sis of brain abscesses. In the absence of surgery, CT can be used to monitor the response to ther-apy of lesions suggestive of cerebral abscesses. The progressive disappearance of brain ab-scesses under antibiotic treatment can be dem-onstrated in this manner.

2.1.4.2 Cerebromeningeal Tuberculosis

Tuberculous meningitis is most common in pat-ients who are immunosuppressed and/or on corticosteroid therapy, and usually leads to quadriventricular hydrocephalus. CT demon-strates abnormal cisternal enhancement in most cases, predominantly in the suprasellar cisterns. Deep cerebral hypodense areas sec-ondary to basal arteritis are less frequent find-ings.
Cerebral tuberculomas are demonstrated by CT as hyperdense cortico-subcortical, paraventric-ular, or brain stem nodules, which can simu-late an intracerebral lymphomatous site.

2.1.4.3 Cerebromeningeal Mycoses

The incidence of cerebromeningeal mycoses is much higher in patients with lymphoma than in the normal population, and can manifest as meningitis, encephalitis, abscesses, and granu-lomas.
Mycotic (fungal) meningitis is generally dem-onstrated by CT as abnormal cisternal en-hancement associated with occasionally exten-sive ventricular dilatation. Such patterns re-semble those of tuberculous meningitis. Mycot-ic granulomas exhibit a variety of CT appear-ances. Multiple small nodules showing ringlike or homogeneous enhancement predominate. Larger, solitary lesions exhibiting homoge-neous or ring enhancement are also possible. Like pyogenic abscesses, mycotic abscesses de-velop in immunodeficient hosts unable to com-bat encephalitic propagation; these ill-defined hypodense cerebral lesions show poorly delim-ited, heterogeneous contrast enhancement without any identifiable ring, and carry a poor prognosis.
Cryptococcosis (torulosis) is a rather frequent complication of HD. Torular meningitis, the most prevalent manifestation, has a lower inci-dence of cisternal enhancement than other types of mycotic meningitis. Granulomas (toru-lomas) and brain abscesses are less frequent.
Nocardiosis occurs fairly frequently in immu-nosuppressed patients; granulomas and multi-ple cerebral abscesses predominate. True acti-nomycoses are actually bacterial infections, and their CT appearances simulate a pyogenic ab-scess or a necrotized tumor.
Cerebral aspergillosis generally develops in im-munosuppressed patients as necrotizing men-ingoencephalitis with a poor prognosis. The deep, poorly defined hypodense patches dem-onstrated by CT either do not enhance at all or enhance heterogeneously. Masses simulating a pyogenic abscess or a cystic tumor are less common. Vascular cerebral lesions are more frequent with aspergillosis than with other types of cerebral mycoses. Aspergillar emboli, generally occurring in the sylvian region, can cause frequently hemorrhagic arterial infarc-tion. More distal arteritis and mycotic arterial aneurysms are also possible, and can lead to in-tracerebral hemorrhage. Cerebral arteriogra-phy is useful for the diagnosis of these vascular lesions.
Cerebral coccidioidomycosis causes extensive basal arachnoiditis with hydrocephalus; the CT appearance is similar to that of tuberculous meningitis.
Cerebral candidiasis usually manifests as nonspecific meningoencephalitis. Granulomas and brain and/or choroid plexus abscesses are rarer.

2.1.4.4 Cerebromeningeal Viroses

Herpetic Encephalitis. It is difficult to make a diagnosis by CT during the first 5 days of evo-lution of this serious form of encephalitis; find-ings are limited to the demonstration of diffuse edematous cerebral swelling with diffuse bilat-

18   D. Gardeur et al.

eral gyriform enhancement. The lesions of herpetic encephalitis typically visible by electroencephalography often appear earlier than the
suggestive CT signs. Unilateral or bilateral temporal or frontotemporobasal hypodense lesions cannot be identified until the end of the
1st week and during the 2nd week of the course
of the disease. They gradually become more
distinct and better circumscribed. Thick gyriform or bandlike enhancements exist at this
stage, and the mass effect on the ventricles increases. CT findings during the 3rd and 4th
weeks of evolution depend on the response to
therapy. When chemotherapy is not administered or is unsuccessful, the temporal hypodense areas continue to spread, the mass effect
becomes stronger, and hemorrhagic disorganization can occur. When treatment proves effective, the cerebral hypodense areas decrease in
size or even disappear, giving way to dilatation
of the temporal horn and the sylvian vallecula.
The sequelae of herpetic encephalitis first become identifiable during the 2nd month of evolution.

Progressive Multifocal Leukoencephalopathy
(PML). PML [59, 105, 140, 291, 343] is a cerebral infection caused by a slow papovavirus
observed almost exclusively in patients with
lymphoma and in immunologically compro-
mised individuals. The CT appearance is characterized by abnormal areas of white matter
hypodensity (Fig. 2.13), reflecting the demyelination characteristic of the pathology. Despite
the denomination "multifocal," these hypodense areas are often monofocal during the
early stages. Hypodense areas are usually noted in the parieto-occipital region, although
frontal, temporal, and capsular sites are also
possible. In a later stage, diffuse areas of hypodensity occur throughout the white matter.
There is generally no mass effect on the ventricular system; on the contrary, the ventricles are
often dilated, owing to progressively worsening
subcortical atrophy. Enhancement is infrequent, although there have been reports of
pseudotumoral lesions during edematous progressive disease.

Subacute Sclerosing Panencephalitis (SSPE).
Described by van Bogaert, SSPE is a slow virus
infection (modified measles virus). Although

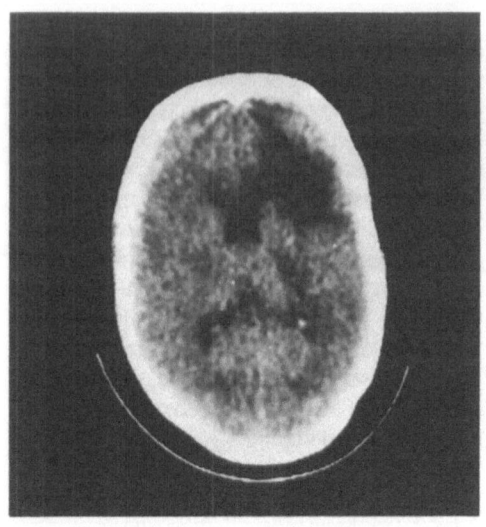

Fig. 2.13. HD in remission. CT showed an abnormal
hypodense area in the frontal white matter, corresponding to progressive multifocal leukoencephalopathy (PML)

usually observed in children and adolescents
several years after a case of measles, SSPE has
also been reported in patients with lymphoma.
In most cases, and especially in forms that
evolve over a period of several years, CT demonstrates progressively increasing ventricular
dilatation indicative of subcortical atrophy. Associated sulcal-cisternal widening is frequent.
Diffuse hypodense areas are fairly common in
the white matter. Symmetrical hypodensities in
the central gray nuclei are rarer, and there is no
abnormal enhancement pattern. During the initial stages, when CT examinations may be com-
pletely normal, electroencephalography is required for diagnosis.

Granulomatous Angiitis with Herpes Zoster Vi-
rus Infection. This pathology is characterized
by diffuse fibrinoid necrosis of the walls of the
cerebral veins and small arteries, and a marked
perivascular inflammatory infiltrate. The viral
origin of granulomatous angiitis is associated
with a herpes zoster infection [193, 246, 627].
Lymphoma patients are often affected. CT
findings usually consist in diffuse bilateral
edematous hypodense lesions with ventricular
and cisternal compression; these lesions are
nonenhancing. Less frequently, more focal hypodense lesions with a mass effect and ische-

mic-appearing enhancement are demonstrated. Carotid arteriography often reveals diffuse distal and segmental lesions of arteritis. PML with herpes zoster virus has been reported in immunosuppressed patients [291], but the relationship between this last pathology and granulomatous angiitis remains to be shown.

2.1.4.5 Parasitoses

Acquired cerebral toxoplasmosis (Fig. 2.14) in the adult almost always occurs in immunodeficient individuals, and especially in patients with lymphoma. Most cases of acquired cerebral toxoplasmosis manifest as brain abscesses or granulomas. Multiple masses prevail (over 70% of cases). Involvement of the central gray nuclei is very common and quite characteristic, but corticomedullary and diffuse white matter lesions also occur. Abnormal enhancement patterns are identifiable in over 75% of cases; homogeneous nodular opacifications; thick, irregular rims; heterogeneous masses; and, more rarely, well-defined rings. The differential diagnosis for focal heterogeneous masses in the central gray nuclei is difficult in cases of AIDS, and brain biopsy is necessary to differentiate a toxoplasmotic abscess from an intracerebral lymphomatous site.

2.1.5 Protocol for Exploration
by Imaging Modalities

Regardless of the type of intracranial complication occurring during the course of a lymphoma, CT should be the first radiological examination. In view of the relative rarity of cerebral manifestations of lymphomas, craniocerebral CT probably need not be included as part of routine staging and surveillance work-ups, but the indications for CT depend on neurologic signs. Systematic cranial CT appears advisable during the course of certain chemotherapy and radiotherapy protocols noted for their aggressivity toward the central nervous system (intrathecal methotrexate, for example).
Radiography of the skull remains indispensable for the exploration of the cephalic osseous structures, but its systematic use is even less necessary than that of CT.

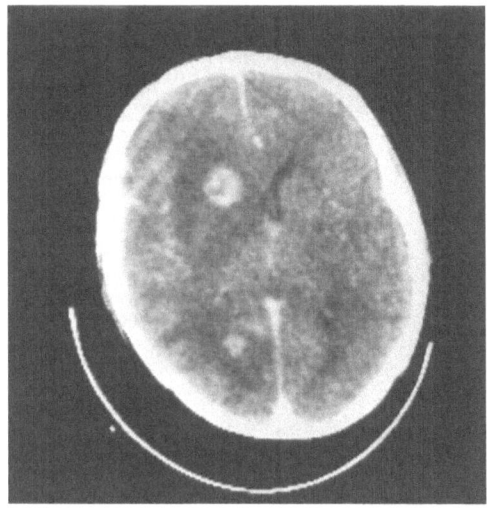

Fig. 2.14. Cerebral toxoplasmosis during HD: hypodense infiltration of right cerebral hemisphere with two areas of enhancement (right occipital and lenticular sites)

Cerebral angiography is only rarely required after CT, for the investigation of certain hemorrhagic lesions or the diagnosis of infectious, tumoral, or radiation angiitis. When surgery is contraindicated, this technique can prove useful for differential diagnosis. Digital angiography is an excellent method for detecting occlusion of the venous sinuses of the dura mater.
Radionuclide brain scans are now indicated only exceptionally for those rare cases of diffuse cerebral lymphoma poorly visualized by CT. By contrast, radionuclide bone scans are still very useful for investigation of the base of the skull and the vertex.

2.2 Intraspinal Lymphoma

2.2.1 Tumoral Infiltration

Epidural sites (Figs. 2.15 and 2.16) account for the majority of tumoral infiltrations [82, 108, 213, 257, 297, 334, 443, 577]. Lymphomatous epiduritis occurs during the course of 0.9%–6.5% of NHL cases, and is a finding in 10%–15% of autopsies for NHL. Tumoral infiltration is secondary to vertebral involvement in 37%–63% of cases of NHL and in nearly all cases of HD. The remaining cases are either

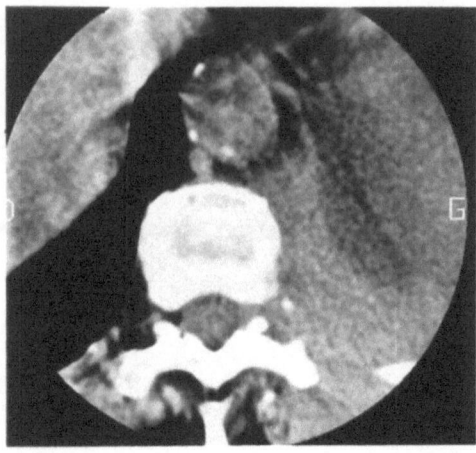

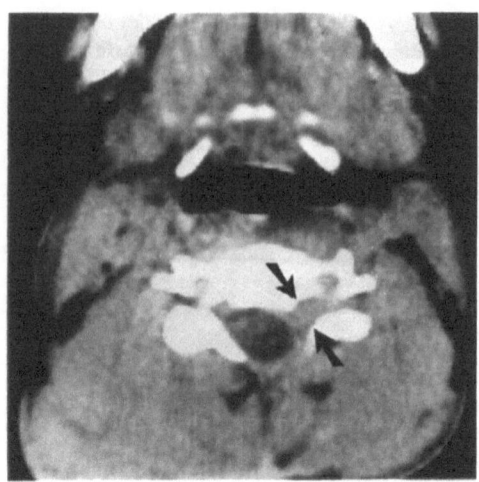

Fig. 2.15. Left paravertebral lymphoma (intraspinal tumor spread through a left intervertebral foramen). The epidural fat is asymmetrical: visible on the *right*, compressed on the *left*

Fig. 2.16. Patient with tonsillar and retroperitoneal NHL: recent onset of left cervicobrachial (C-3, C-4, C-5) neuralgia. CT demonstrated an abnormal left laterocervical epidural mass near and within the intervertebral foramina *(arrows)*

primary, or secondary to infiltration of a paravertebral mass.

2.2.1.1 Histopathologic Mechanisms

Various mechanisms can cause neurologic involvement:

- Primary epidural or, more rarely, subarachnoid lymphomatous sites
- Contiguous extension from a vertebral bone lesion or from a paravertebral soft-tissue tumor, by spread through the intervertebral foramina
- Ischemic myelomalacia resulting from vascular compression, especially involving Adamkiewicz's artery
- Intramedullary extension

2.2.1.2 Clinical Picture and Radiological Exploration

Lymphomatous epiduritis generally affects the dorsal spinal cord (51%–91% of cases); lumbar (9%–36%), cervical (0%–24%), and sacral (0%–12%) disease sites are much less frequent.

Clinical symptoms are varied (Table 2.1). Radiography of the spine is indicated for initial investigations. Complementary studies depend on the clinical context (degree of neurosurgical urgency, localizing signs of the lesion) and whether or not bone lesions are detected on standard spinal films. Supplementary information can be obtained by CT of the spine, myelography with iodized oil (Lipiodol) or metrizamide (Amipaque), and gas myelography.

When lesions are demonstrated clinically or radiologically, *CT* should be performed first, since scans generally suffice for decisions as to the advisability of neurosurgery or radiotherapy. CT demonstrates lymphomatous epiduritis as a soft-tissue dense mass that obliterates the epidural fat and compresses the dural sac [268, 508]. These tumors usually enhance in an intense, homogeneous manner; the hyperdense tumor is thus readily distinguished from the compressed dural sac. For epiduritis secondary to vertebral bone lesions, CT accurately visualizes the bone lysis adjacent to the epidural mass. In other cases, CT reveals spread of an epidural mass toward one or more intervertebral foramina, occasionally with lesion extension to the paravertebral soft tissues. In this last type of tumoral spread, the epidural site is generally lateral or posterolateral. Centromedullary enhancement secondary to tumoral infiltration or to ischemic myelomalacia is a rare finding. Medullary arteriography is usually not justified to visualize compression of Adamkiewicz's artery.

When there are no clinical localizing signs and/or when CT cannot be performed immediately, *myelography* is indicated. For certain authors, emergency diagnosis of tumoral epiduritis remains one of the last indications for iodized oil myelography. Other authors prefer water-soluble contrast agents, which provide better tumor definition, but these products involve a greater risk of neurologic aggravation and more side effects. Delayed films cannot be obtained with water-soluble agents, and there is no residual product which would allow ulterior surveillance of the course of the disease. Double-contrast myelography provides better delineation of the superior and inferior margins of the tumor. In addition to the use of lumbar and suboccipital punctures for determination of the extent of the tumor in cases of complete blockage, complementary injection of 5 ml of air has recently been suggested during iodized oil myelography so that the product can circumnavigate a complete block [334].

Myelographic findings depend on the site of epidural involvement and the degree of blockage. Complete blocks are noted in 46%–75% of iodized oil myelographies, but are less frequent in myelography with water-soluble contrast agents and after the complementary injection of air. The site of obstruction to the flow of contrast product which is due to epidural involvement is usually visualized as an irregular lesion with a saw-toothed or comb-teeth appearance. Certain primary epidural tumors are associated with multiple, irregular forms with a serpiginous appearance. In certain less extensive cases of epidural involvement, and especially in lateral or posterolateral sites, myelography with water-soluble products demonstrates extrinsic compression of the dural sac as a large, scalloped indentation.

After surgery (laminectomy) and/or radiotherapy, CT generally suffices for follow-up evaluation of tumor size. When iodized oil has been left in place, appropriate patient mobilization allows new studies.

2.2.2 Iatrogenic Pathologies

Abnormal enhancement of the spinal cord has been reported several months or years after abdominal or thoracic radiotherapy [495], apparently owing to radiation injuries of the blood-nerve tissue barrier, similar to the lesions of cerebral radionecrosis.

Medullary atrophy is the most frequent complication of spinal cord irradiation. While medullary atrophy in the cervical region can generally be diagnosed by CT, thoracic sites occasionally require supplementary myelographic studies.

Medullary demyelination secondary to intrathecal injection of methotrexate [132] cannot currently be visualized by CT. Magnetic resonance imaging (MRI) may provide better information in the future; MRI will also probably allow three-dimensional visualization of epidural lymphomatous involvement and the relationships of these lesions with the spinal cord, thereby obviating the need for intrathecal injection of contrast medium.

3 Orbital Lymphomas

E. A. CABANIS, J. TAMRAZ, M.-L. JABLON, AND M.-T. IBA-ZIZEN

Orbital lymphomas account for nearly 10% of all expansile lesions of the orbit, a frequency which places them just after orbital hemangiomas and, especially, granulomas, the most frequent pathology, which includes both thyroid ophthalmopathies and the nosologically more problematical inflammatory pseudotumors [165, 269, 307]. The incidence of orbital lymphomas is much lower in children, having been estimated at approximately 1% [273, 274, 309]. In fact, the great majority of these lymphoproliferative orbital syndromes are encountered in adults; the few exceptions concern mainly Burkitt's lymphoma, a lymphoblastic form principally affecting children. Hodgkin's disease (HD) rarely involves the orbit. The causal element of most non-Hodgkin's lymphomas (NHL) is B-lymphocyte proliferation [317, 487, 516, 678].

Rappaport's classification was selected from the many available staging systems for use in the present report on 22 cases of histologically confirmed orbital lymphomas, all of which were analyzed by computed tomography (CT) at the Centre National d'Ophtalmologie des XV-XX (Paris). Since standard roentgenography and its ultrasound correlations generally provide little diagnostic information in such cases, these two preliminary diagnostic approaches have been voluntarily excluded from the present discussion (Fig. 3.1).

3.1 Materials and Methods

Between 1978 and 1984, nearly 5000 of the 22 000 patients examined by CT in our neuroradiology department presented with neuroophthalmologic symptoms. Following an initial selection of 50 hematological cases, the study was finally restricted to NHL of the orbit. A total of 22 clinically and radiologically exploitable

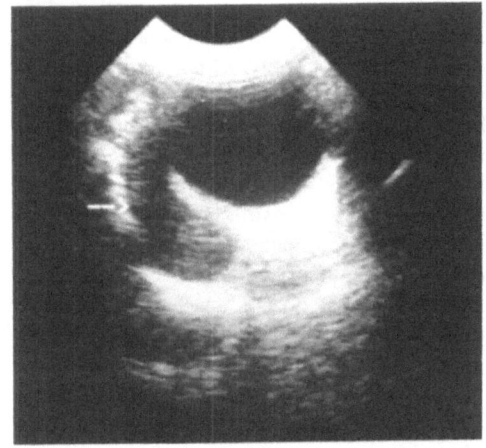

Fig. 3.1. Sonogram of an intraorbital lymphoma

cases were obtained, all with histopathological confirmation.

The study population consisted of 21 adults (13 women, 8 men) aged 45-80 years and one 2-year-old child. Eighteen of the patients were over 50 years of age at the time of CT scanning, and 70% of them were between 50 and 60 years.

A strict procedure was followed for the investigation of all 22 patients. The orbitocephalic plane of incidence corresponded to the neuro-ocular plane, defined as the CT section plane that passes successively through the two lens hyperdensities, the heads of the two optic nerves, and finally the optic canals in the primary position of gaze. The importance of this neuro-ocular plane no longer needs to be demonstrated, as most authors consider it the most appropriate for analysis of the anterior optic pathways and their orbital environment, both for axial and for coronal and sagittal views following three-dimensional reconstruction. Moreover, the precision of the landmarks in this reference plane allows assessment of the evolution of lesions, which is indispensable for differential diagnosis and the evaluation of response to therapeutic tests. Oculo-orbital biometry, used to define the degree of exophthalmos (grades I–III), and dynamic tests of lateral globe excursion supplemented the CT scans obtained for all 22 patients before and after intravenous injection of an iodinated contrast medium. A standard six-projection radiographic survey completed investigations.

3.2 Results and Discussion

The clinical presenting manifestations of NHL were ophthalmologic in almost two-thirds of the cases. In the remaining patients, the orbital and adnexal sites corresponded to extranodal dissemination of a previously diagnosed malignant lymphoma. The interval between initial diagnosis and the development of ophthalmologic symptoms was around 2 years. CT was always performed in the month following the appearance of the clinical signs. The major presenting symptoms were orbitopalpebral swelling (12 cases), with (10 cases) or without (2 cases) associated exophthalmos, and, less frequently, impaired ocular motility which did or did not cause diplopia (4 cases). Clinical examination detected adenopathies in 9 cases; a pulmonary or mediastinal disease site in 5 cases; subcutaneous nodules in 2 cases; and 1 renal tumor, 1 parotid tumor, and 1 breast tumor. The anatomical distribution of these lesions and the consequent swelling were well correlated with anatomical data which situate the orbital lymphatics at the level of the conjunctivae and the eyelids and in the lacrimal glands under normal conditions. This explains why our series revealed certain sites of predilection for orbital lymphomas, corresponding to complaints by patients of swelling of the upper eyelid and outer canthal regions (9 cases) or of the lower eyelid (3 cases). Subcutaneous tumors were usually firm, smooth, nonpainful, and relatively movable on palpation (Table 3.1).

CT confirmed the lacrimal, superior temporal compartment (10 cases) as the *predominant site* of lymphoid tumors. One of these cases was associated with discrete osseous erosion of the lateral orbital wall. Involvement was primarily located in the intraconal orbital fat and the orbital apex in three cases, and in the inferior nasal compartment in three other cases. Of these 16 patients, 3 had *bilateral lesions*. The right orbit was involved in ten cases, the left orbit in nine cases. Solitary *intraconal* lesions occurred in four patients. The extraconal compartments were affected in six cases, five of which exhibited extension into the intraconal compartment. Three patients had a large retroscleral tumor, but no deformation of the posterior part of the globe. Muscle infiltration was noted in at least two cases. Three patients had more diffuse involvement, with considerably increased volumes of intraorbital fat; although there was no increase in muscle cone volume, modification of the attenuation coefficient of the orbital fat produced a pseudo-de Saint Yves syndrome. The CT appearance of lesions included a *spontaneous hyperdensity* which was moderately enhanced on postcontrast scans in most cases. Nevertheless, in three cases, the relatively strong enhancement and morphological characteristics of the tumor, plus the presence of ocular inflammatory signs, led us to entertain the possibility of an inflammatory orbital pseudotumor. The clinical course, absence of a frank response to corticosteroid testing, and serial CT scans eventually caused us to reject this last hypothesis (Table 3.2).

The *histopathological distribution* of these orbital lymphomas according to the Rappaport classification [515], with its widely acknowledged clinical and prognostic value, included ten cases of mixed NHL (five nodular, five diffuse), six cases of well-differentiated lymphocytic NHL (lymphocytosarcoma), two cases of poorly differentiated lymphocytic NHL (lymphoblastosarcoma), three cases of histiocytic NHL (reticulosarcoma), and one case of undifferentiated NHL (Burkitt). In analyzing the significance of this distribution, it must be remembered that the study was deliberately limited to NHL, and that benign and intermediate lymphoid hyperplasias were excluded. Of the 22 cases retained, 17 were diffuse and 5 were nodular.

Table 3.1. Focal and general clinical signs

Patient	Sex	Age	Oculo-orbital clinical symptoms	Systemic signs
1	F	66	Dry-eye syndrome RO Lobular masses: left superior and inferior palpebral folds Exophthalmos RO (21 mm) Impaired ocular motility Intracranial bruit	Adenopathies Elevated sedimentation rate Pneumopathy
2	M	50	Tearing Movable swelling of lower right eyelid along the orbital rim	
3	M	72	Left orbital cyst requiring subtotal resection	Iliac adenopathies
4	F	60	Left orbital swelling, smooth, nonpainful, freely movable, lacrimal location	Supraclavicular adenopathies
5	F	44	Thin, reddish conjunctival swelling of the lower left eyelid	Inguinal adenopathies
6	F	52	Eyelid edema Ptosis Well-defined, freely movable, nonpainful swelling, lacrimal location	Pretragal adenopathies
7	F	64	Left conjunctival hyperemia Band keratopathy Right and left suprapalpebral nodules Lacrimal swelling Exophthalmos LO, nonaxile, nonpainful	
8	M	71	Horizontal diplopia (right V nerve) Blindness RO Horner's syndrome Right V and right VII nerves	
9	F	64	Subconjunctival hemorrhage and hyphema RO	Subcutaneous nodules
10	M	54	Ptosis Diplopia (III and IV nerves) Discrete exophthalmos	Adenopathies
11	F	46	Left chemosis Left exophthalmos, nonaxile, irreducible, nonpainful	

Table 3.1 *(continued)*

Patient	Sex	Age	Oculo-orbital clinical symptoms	Systemic signs
12	F	66	Swelling of upper right eyelid, nonpainful, firm, freely movable External palpebral nodules	Left parotid swelling No adenopathy
13	F	58	Orbitopalpebral swelling, exophthalmos, axile, nonpainful, irreducible Upper eyelid retraction RO/LO	Cervical, axillary and inguinal adenopathies Renal tumor
14	F	72	Swelling of upper right eyelid Moderate exophthalmos RO/LO	Adenopathies Subcutaneous nodules
15	F	60	Intermittent diplopia Edema of lower right eyelid Papilledema RO Exophthalmos RO	
16	M	36	Tearing RO Swelling of the upper cul-de-sac Pain Visual loss RO	
17	F	61	Exophthalmos LO Papilledema LO Inferior nasal quadrantanopia LO Visual acuity LO 2/20 Left ptosis and left V nerves	
18	M	60	Chemosis LO Exophthalmos RO Right V, left peripheral VII nerve	Pleurisy Mediastinal adenopathies (lymphoma)
19	F	81	Exophthalmos RO, nonaxile Superotemporal orbital swelling	Pneumopathy Breast tumor
20	M	77	Lower right subpalpebral swelling, firm, freely movable	
21	M	2	Exophthalmos LO, axile, irreducible Orbitopalpebral swelling	
22	M	60	Diplopia Retrobulbar optic neuritis Right peripheral VII nerve	

RO, right orbit; *LO*, left orbit

Table 3.2. CT-histopathology correlations

Patient	CT features	Histopathological diagnosis
1	SOL of the left medial rectus muscle and right inferior rectus muscle (inferior nasal compartment) Hyperdensity with subcutaneous outer canthal infiltration (left > right) Exophthalmos RO, axial (3 mm)	Diffuse well-differentiated lymphoma (node biopsy)
2	Exophthalmos RO/LO (RO > LO), grade II then grade III (in 2 years) Increased volume of orbital fat (de Saint Yves syndrome)	Diffuse, well-differentiated lymphoma (orbital fat biopsy) Thyrotropin-releasing hormone (test −)
3	Extraconal, left inferior nasal SOL with mass effect on the left ethmoid plate and left ocular globe	Mixed nodular lymphoma (tumor biopsy) (marrow biopsy + or −)
4	Intra- and extraconal SOL, lacrimal superior temporal compartment, hyperdense plus contrast enhancement No mass effect on the ocular globe Discrete lysis of lateral orbital wall Subcutaneous outer canthal infiltration	Mixed nodular lymphoma (tumor biopsy) (marrow biopsy +)
5	Normal appearance	Mixed nodular lymphoma (conjunctival biopsy)
6	Enlargement of right lacrimal gland Appearance compatible with an inflammatory pseudotumor (recurrence of SOL on successive examinations)	Mixed nodular lymphoma (node biopsy)
7	Left intra- and extraconal SOL: hyperdense plus enhancement after i.v. injection of contrast medium Location: retroscleral LO, outer canthus and left inferior orbit (nasal compartment) Infiltration of left inferior rectus muscle Left and right pretragal node Lymphoma or inflammatory pseudotumor	Diffuse, well-differentiated lymphoma (cutaneous nodule biopsy)
8	Intraconal SOL of apex of RO Possible infiltration of lateral rectus muscles and inferior rectus muscles Juxtacanalicular portion of right optic nerve enveloped by the mass Extension: sphenoidal fissure	Diffuse, well-differentiated lymphoma (marrow biopsy)
9	Normal appearance	Diffuse, poorly differentiated, lymphocytic NHL (subcutaneous nodule biopsy)
10	No SOL Bilateral exophthalmos, grade I de Saint-Yves syndrome	Diffuse, well-differentiated NHL (node biopsy)
11	Intra- and extraconal SOL, retro- and suprascleral LO plus development in superior temporal compartment (predominantly lacrimal) Hyperdense Right lateral rectus muscle and superior rectus muscle enveloped by the mass Exophthalmos LO, grade II Lymphoma or inflammatory pseudotumor	Mixed nodular lymphoma

Table 3.2 *(continued)*

Patient	CT features	Histopathological diagnosis
12	Rounded, cystic, subcutaneous SOLs, outer canthal location: lacrimal origin? No mass effect on the ocular globes	Diffuse, well-differentiated lymphoma (salivary gland biopsy) (marrow biopsy +)
13	Right and left SOL, intra- and extraconal Right: superior orbital and temporal SOL; superior rectus muscle and lateral rectus muscle invaded; retro- and suprascleral RO extension Left: superior temporal extraconal SOL plus infiltration of superior rectus muscle, lateral rectus muscle and outer canthal region; internal margin of SOL irregular; exophthalmos grade II	Diffuse mixed lymphoma (node biopsy)
14	Extraconal SOL, right suprascleral and anterior superolateral Lacrimal location No mass effect on RO Exophthalmos RO	Diffuse mixed lymphoma (node biopsy)
15	Intraconal right retrobulbar SOL, hyperdense, contrast-enhanced Exophthalmos grade II	Diffuse mixed lymphoma (orbital tumor biopsy) (marrow biopsy +)
16	Relative RO exophthalmos No intraorbital SOL	Diffuse mixed lymphoma (conjunctival biopsy)
17	Left, juxta-apical intraconal SOL, hyperdense	Diffuse mixed lymphoma (orbital tumor biopsy)
18	Bilateral exophthalmos owing to increased orbital fat volume Diffuse, relative hyperdensity of orbital fat de Saint-Yves syndrome	Diffuse, poorly-differentiated lymphoma (pleural biopsy) (marrow biopsy +)
19	Intra- and extraconal SOL, lacrimal superolateral location, hyperdense plus enhancement after i.v. injection of contrast-medium Exophthalmos, nonaxile, RO displaced inward	Diffuse histiocytic lymphoma (breast nodule biopsy)
20	Inferior intraconal SOL, right infraocular Well-delimited, inferior, and jugal palpebral extension RO displaced upward, no scleral deformation	Diffuse histiocytic lymphoma (orbital tumor biopsy)
21	Extraconal superolateral orbital SOL; lacrimal and outer canthal location; hyperdense plus enhancement after i.v. injection of contrast medium No mass effect on LO No bony involvement of lateral wall Infiltration of anterior portion of lateral rectus muscle	Diffuse histiocytic lymphoma (orbital tumor biopsy)
22	Increased caliber of intraorbital portion of right optic nerve, along the posterior optic cup of the ocular globe Adjacent localized scleral thickening, hyperdense plus enhancement after i.v. injection of contrast medium	Diffuse poorly differentiated lymphoma (Burkitt) (marrow biopsy)

SOL, space-occupying lesion; *RO*, right orbit; *LO*, left orbit

3.3. Conclusion

Orbital lymphomas are a relatively rare phenomenon, accounting for only 3% of the orbital tumors in our series. In the majority of cases they occur late in adult life (average 58 years). The main clinical symptoms include a nonpainful, orbitopalpebral mass, especially superior (55% of cases); exophthalmos (45%); and impaired ocular motility (less than 25%). Ophthalmologic manifestations were the initial signs of disease in nearly 60% of cases. CT examination is thus essential for optimum patient management, as it can confirm presumed cases of oculo-orbital malignant lymphoma.

The differential diagnoses, in order of frequency, include lacrimal or uveal scleral inflammatory pseudotumors, perioptic infiltrating processes of other natures and, in certain cases, even endocrinelike ophthalmopathies causing a solitary and progressive increase in the volume of intraorbital fat.

Positive diagnosis rests on clinical findings and CT features [308, 619, 670] (Figs. 3.2–3.9).

Characteristic CT features include (a) hyperdense homogeneous lesions only slightly enhanced by contrast media (four-fifths of cases); (b) well-defined margins at contact with the tunica of the nondeformed globe and orbital cavity, in rare instances with bone erosion (one-

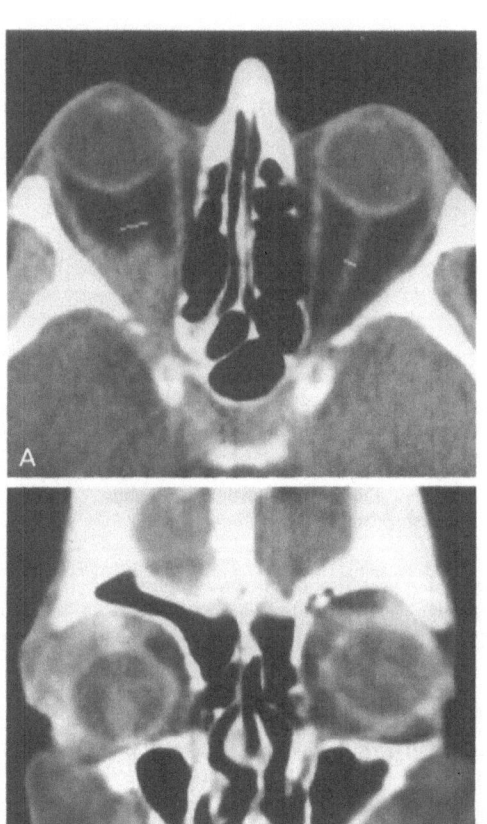

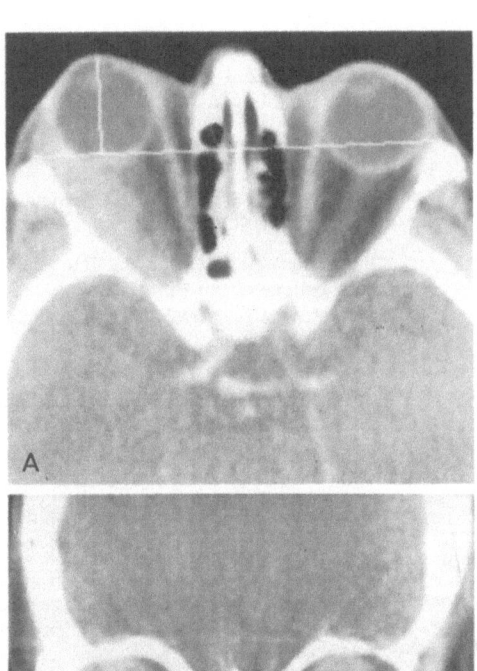

Fig. 3.2 A, B. Case no. 6 (56-year-old woman). **A** Right extraconal superolateral space-occupying lesion: hyperdense and homogeneous; **B** discrete downward displacement of the globe

Fig. 3.3 A, B. Case no. 13 (58-year-old woman). Right and left superior temporal space-occupying lesion indissociable from the affected oculometer muscles, with bilateral exophthalmos. **A** From above; **B** frontal view

tenth of cases); (c) irregular appearance of retrobulbar intraconal extensions; (d) predominantly temporal and/or preseptal extraconal sites; (e) usually negative or nonspecific findings for examinations of conjunctival and palpebral lesions; and (f) no morphological features linked to the histological type.

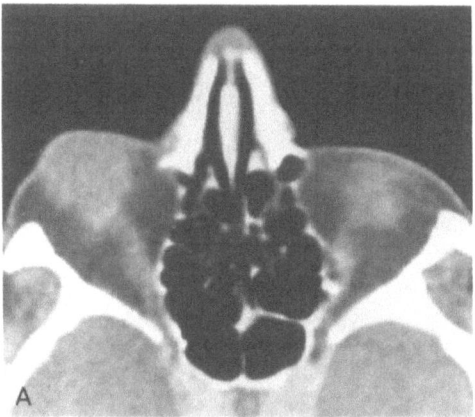

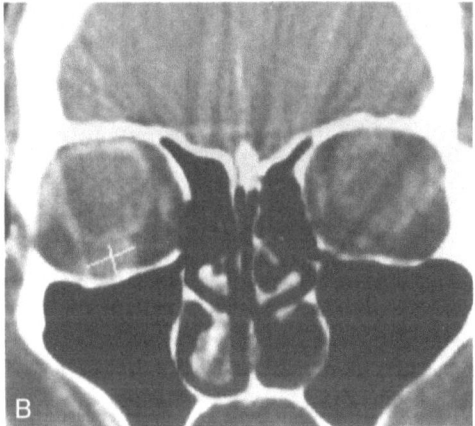

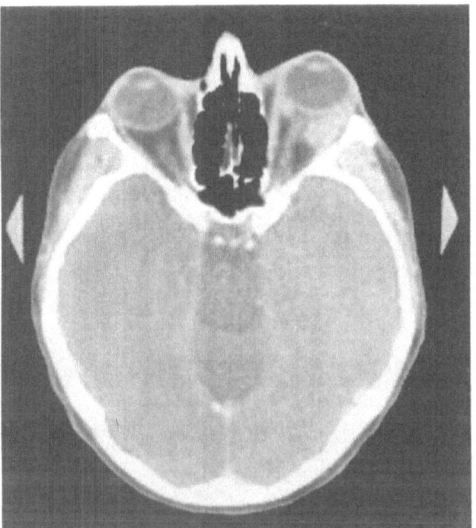

Fig. 3.4. Case no. 11 (46-year-old woman). Left intra- and extraconal space-occupying lesion developing retrosclerally, preserving the head of the optic nerve. The hyperdense, homogeneous lesion infiltrates the lacrimal gland, and there is left exophthalmos

Fig. 3.5 A, B. Case no. 20 (72-year-old man). Right inferior orbital space-occupying lesion indissociable from the inferior rectus muscle, poorly visible in the axial plane (A), better seen in the frontal view (B). There is exophthalmos, and the globe is displaced upward

Fig. 3.6. Case no. 3 (72-year-old man). Left inferior ▷ nasal space-occupying lesion along nasolacrimal duct, preserving the inferior rectus muscle close to the globe

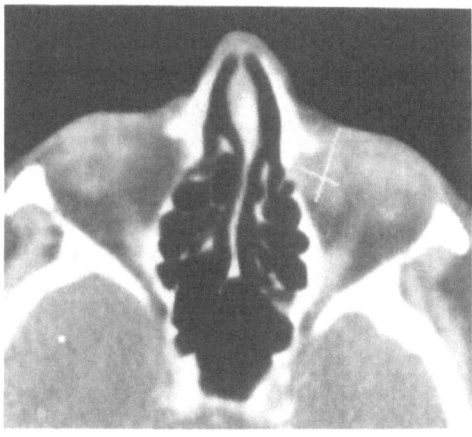

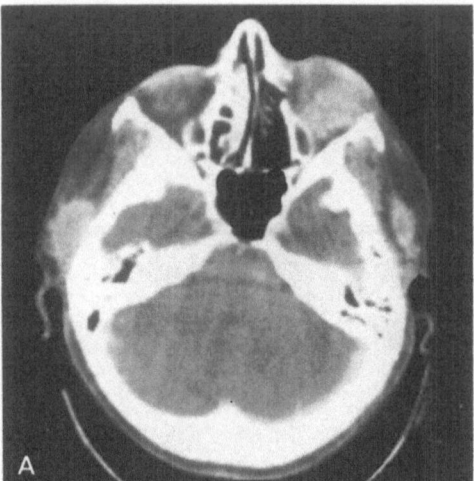

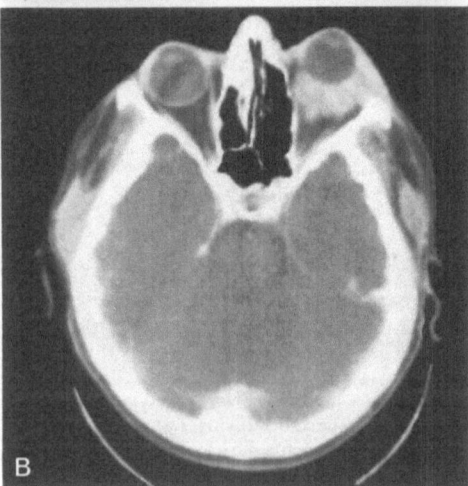

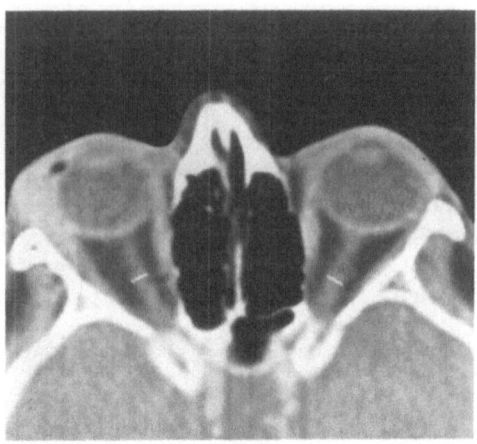

Fig. 3.8. Case no. 8 (71-year-old man). Right intraconal space-occupying lesion invading the apex and extending to the sphenoidal fissure. Mass effect on the lateral rectus muscle indissociable from the lesion. Note the asymmetry of the optic nerves: *right*, enlarged; *left*, atrophic

Fig. 3.7 A, B. Case no. 7 (64-year-old woman). Left extraconal, intraconal retroscleral space-occupying lesion, with bilateral infiltration of pretragal nodes. **B** *CT* scan taken 1 cm above **A**

Fig. 3.9. Case no. 18 (60-year-old man). Enlargement ▷ and infiltration of the right optic nerve, with predominantly right bilateral exophthalmos owing to increased orbital fat

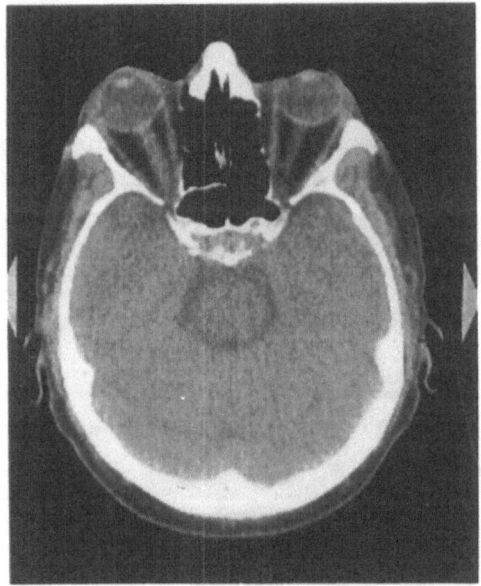

4 Lymphomas of the Face and Neck

J.-N. Bruneton, P. Kerboul, and F. Denis

Lymphomas of the face and neck encompass lymphomatous processes affecting Waldeyer's ring, the facial structures, the thyroid gland, the salivary glands, cervical lymph nodes, the larynx, and the ear. Lymphomas of these sites are fairly common, accounting for 15% of all extranodal non-Hodgkin's lymphomas (NHL) for Freeman [212]. Extranodal sites almost always correspond to NHL, whereas adenopathies are the most frequent manifestation of cervicofacial Hodgkin's disease (HD). This situation is reflected in the fact that Ennuyer's 1961 literature review [187] cited only 33 extranodal sites of HD. HD of the face and neck is thus essentially a nodal pathology; NHL usually presents as an extranodal cervicofacial lesion.

Men are affected more often than women [74, 607], and patients are on average over 50 years of age. Three clinical situations are possible:

In most cases, the disease is heralded by functional ear, nose, and throat manifestations which lead to specialized investigations and the consequent diagnosis of lymphoma, plus a pretherapy work-up.

In cases of solitary cervical adenopathies, systematic clinical examination of the head and neck regions results in diagnosis.

Less frequently, cervicofacial exploration is performed as part of a work-up for generalized lymphoma.

Histologically, diffuse disease is the most prevalent form of NHL [661]. The prognosis is generally related to the histological type. Well-differentiated lymphocytic disease has a very good prognosis [200], whereas associations of cervical adenopathies and visceral involvement have a poor outlook.

4.1 Waldeyer's Ring

Waldeyer's ring is formed by the tonsils, the nasopharynx, the base of the tongue, the posterior pharyngeal wall, and the palate. The highest incidences of lymphoma occur in the first three anatomical sites. Although lesions are often solitary, multiple foci are present in 10%–16% of cases [13, 74, 661]. Waldeyer's ring is the most frequent site of cervicofacial NHL; it is only rarely affected by HD [13, 28]. The reported incidence of involvement of Waldeyer's ring in cervicofacial NHL varies from 49% to 72% of cases [74, 93, 200, 661]. Associated cervical adenopathies are present in slightly under half of all patients, retroperitoneal nodes exist in one-third of cases, and gastrointestinal sites, especially in the stomach, are involved in one-fifth of cases [28]. Diffuse forms are the most prevalent histological type; nodular forms are exceptional [28, 74].

The mean prognosis for NHL is 75%–90% survival at 5 years for localized disease, and 16%–50% survival at 5 years when there are adenopathies [200]. These figures rise to 94% survival at 3 years for well-differentiated lymphocytic forms, but drop to only 58% at 3 years for histiocytic forms [200]. The prognosis for HD stages I and II is 94%–100%, and 76% for stages III or IV [186].

Recurrences generally occur within 2 years, usually as extranodal involvement of the gastrointestinal tract or of the bones [28, 74]. The site with the worst prognosis remains the subject of controversy; certain authors feel tonsillar lesions have the worst outcome [200, 661], but others have singled out the rhinopharynx [74].

The tonsil, the main site in Waldeyer's ring, accounts for less than 10% of all NHL [212], but for 51%–53.3% of cervicofacial NHL [607, 642]. Within Waldeyer's ring itself, tonsillar lesions are responsible for 33%–72% of cases [28, 74, 93, 661]. NHL represents between 2% and 41.6% of all tonsillar malignancies [186, 322, 607, 640]. HD of the tonsil is rare (18 cases in the 1961 review by Ennuyer [187]).

Clinical symptoms are often of a pharyngeal nature (unilateral pharyngeal discomfort, sore throat, unilateral dysphagia) [74, 607]. In other instances, examination is prompted by the discovery of cervical adenopathies. Of variable size, the tumor is usually firm, nonpainful and covered by a purplish-blue mucosa. Less suggestive appearances include ulcerating or infiltrating lesions or, on the contrary, very superficial lesions. Adenopathies are present in 53%–65% of cases [607, 642] (Fig. 4.1).

The nasopharynx is the site of less than 3% of all primary extranodal NHL [212], and the location of 18.5%–32.5% of cases of NHL in Waldeyer's ring [13, 28, 93, 661]. NHL is responsible for 1.2%–43.9% of all malignant tumors of the nasopharynx [459, 613, 671]. HD of the nasopharynx is rare [13]. Lesions are generally solitary, although there may be concomitant lymphomatous tonsillar lesions [28].

Clinical features include unilateral or bilateral nasal obstruction and loss of hearing. Clinical examination can detect a soft, hemorrhagic mass on the roof of the cavum; diffuse involvement is also possible. In contrast to tonsillar sites, adenopathies are rare.

The *base of the tongue* is the third most frequent site of lymphomas in Waldeyer's ring, accounting for 2.7%–18% of cases [28, 93, 661]. NHL is the cause of 1.2%–4.6% of all tongue malignancies [210, 372]. Clinical symptoms include a foreign body sensation, dysphagia, and cervical adenopathies.

The various imaging techniques play the same role for the investigation of lymphomas in Waldeyer's ring as for the investigation of carcinomas. CT in particular is especially valuable for analysis of the cavum, allowing easy lesion staging and detection of the bone involvement which can appear during the late stages of the disease; this in turn facilitates follow-up of patients (Figs. 4.2–4.4).

Transverse CT scans do not always allow very accurate exploration of the base of the tongue or the tonsils, especially if dental artifacts are present during initial work-up. Ultrasonography performed using a submental approach is

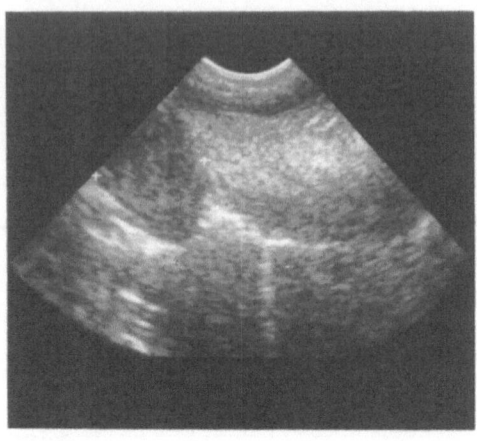

Fig. 4.1. Tonsillar NHL (sonogram obtained with a sagittal submental approach: well-limited, 26-mm-diameter hypoechoic lesion). The base of the tongue located in front appears homogeneous and more echogenic

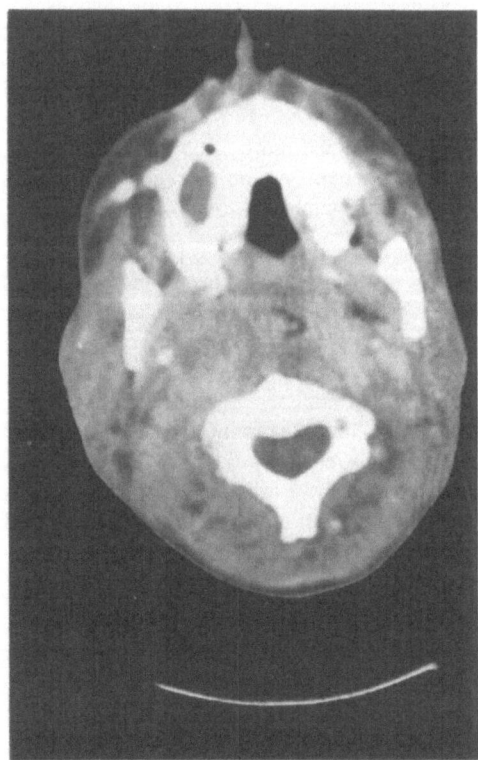

Fig. 4.2. NHL of the cavum

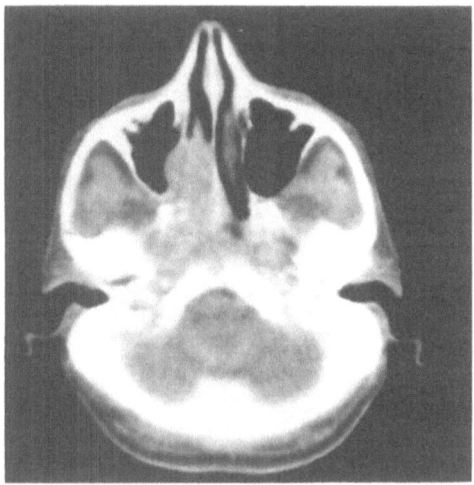

Fig. 4.3. NHL of the nasopharynx

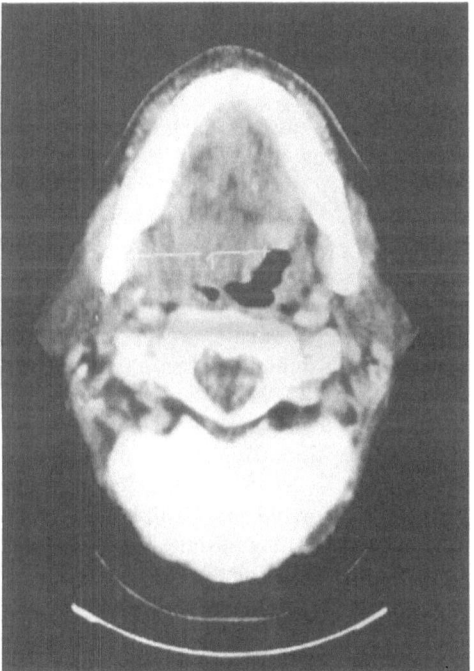

Fig. 4.4. NHL of the base of the tongue. *Line 1*, 5 cm

helpful in such cases to delineate tumor size and to assess response to treatment.

The frequency of associated retroperitoneal involvement underlines the importance of CT exploration of the thorax and abdomen [28, 74]. Likewise, the risk of intranodal recurrence justifies both gastrointestinal studies and scintigraphy aimed at detecting any bone involvement.

4.2 Facial Structures

The facial structures are the second most frequent site of NHL after Waldeyer's ring, representing 7%-30% of NHL sites [74, 93, 403]. NHL accounts for 14.5%-25% of all malignant tumors of the facial structures. There is a discrete male predominance (sex ratio 1.3). Clinically, unilateral nasal obstruction is usually associated with asymmetrical facial swelling [643], and 24% of patients present with cervical adenopathies [643]. Examination reveals a granular tumor filling the nasal cavity. The prognosis for these hemorrhagic, nonulcerating polypoid growths is better than for lymphomas of Waldeyer's ring, as the survival rate at 5 years is 80% [200]. Radiological study generally demonstrates the internal septum of the maxillary sinus as an irregular, homogeneous opacity. Occasionally, complete opacification of the sinuses suggests chronic maxillary sinusitis [370]. Bone lysis can occur with large lesions. Lesions can regress with therapy, giving way to sequelar thickening and recalcification of previously lytic bone lesions (Figs. 4.5–4.7).

4.3 Thyroid Gland

Primary lymphomas of the thyroid gland are very rare, representing only 0.29% of all lymphomas and 2.5% of all extranodal forms [212]. NHL predominates, accounting for 92.5%-97.8% of all thyroid lymphomas [432, 664]. These figures underscore the extreme rarity of primary HD of the thyroid gland. Fewer than 20 cases of thyroid HD have been published in the literature worldwide [1, 231, 432], whereas over 250 reports were found concerning NHL, which is responsible for 3%-4% of all thyroid cancers [86, 95, 568]. Owing to the

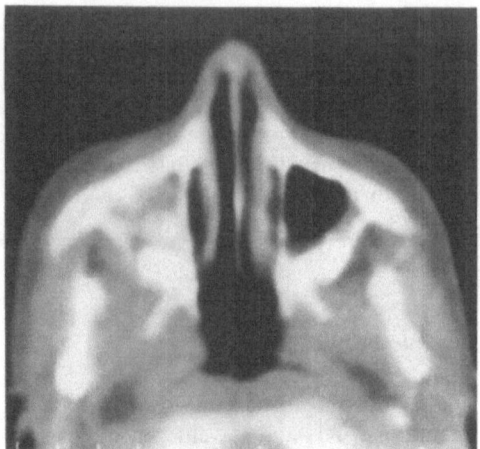

Fig. 4.5. NHL of the right maxillary sinus

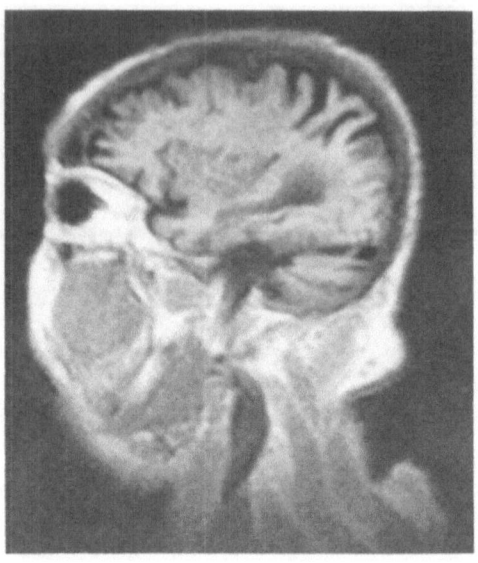

Fig. 4.7. NHL of the right maxillary sinus seen by magnetic resonance imaging (MRI): sagittal view

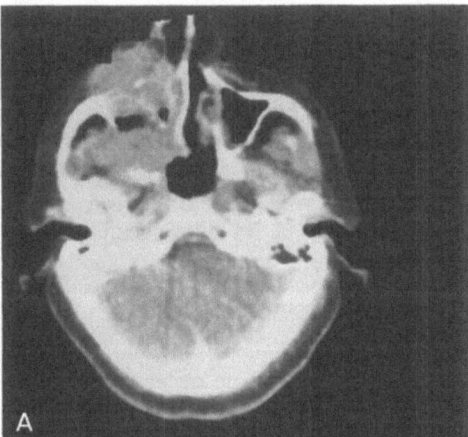

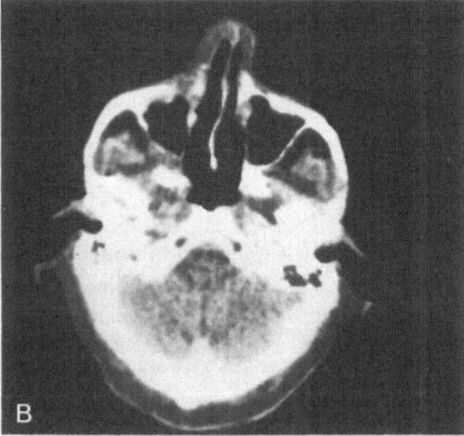

Fig. 4.6 A, B. NHL of the right maxillary sinus. A Before and B 3 months after treatment

rarity of primary thyroid HD, the greater part of the following discussion is given over to NHL.

Histology studies have demonstrated the predominance of histiocytic types, especially in diffuse forms [86]. While radiotherapy has been cited as a predisposing factor on rare occasions [47], 10.9%–26.7% of cases are reportedly associated with Hashimoto's disease (struma lymphomatosa) [432, 571, 664]. This association, which carries a good prognosis, raises the possibility of transition from a benign process to lymphoma [337, 390, 527, 604].

The course of thyroid gland lymphomas can involve spread to the gastrointestinal tract, and the incidence of gastrointestinal lesions is higher with thyroid lymphomas than with other primary lymphomas [641, 664]. Both localized and diffuse forms can extend beyond the capsule. The main diagnostic problem is differentiation from anaplastic small-cell carcinoma [664]. Clinically, the typical patient is an elderly woman with diffuse or localized swelling of the neck, often of recent onset. Dysphagia is not uncommon in diffuse disease [664]. The prognosis for primary NHL of the thyroid gland varies from 48%–54% survival at 5 years [86, 212] to only 25% at 10 years, and thus seems less favorable than for other thyroid cancers.

Radionuclide studies demonstrate thyroid lymphomas as cold nodules in the nonfunctioning lobes [125]. Although ultrasound cannot specify the nature of lesions, there are three distinct sonographic patterns [78]:

Solitary nodules, oval, strongly hypoechoic lesions, occasionally resemble cysts, but there are always a few distal echoes which rule out this hypothesis. The differential diagnosis is a necrotized adenoma (Figs. 4.8 and 4.9).

Diffuse heterogenic lesions with a complex echo pattern owing to the coexistence of lymphomatous zones and uninvolved tissue. Enlargement of the various thyroid diameters and the presence of multiple hypoechoic nodules on sonograms can suggest multinodular goiter. The common diagnosis for rapidly growing lesions is cancer. Ultrasound is useful for detecting involvement of the surrounding soft tissues, and muscles in particular. Any associated cervical adenopathies are also readily visualized.

Diffuse hypertrophic forms with a normal echostructure. Lesions of this type have been observed in clinically evident multiorgan disease. Return to normal of glandular volume under chemotherapy, along with regression of other lymphomatous sites, provides retrospective proof of thyroid involvement.

Mention must also be made of the notable frequency of thyroid complications (hypothyroidism and/or thyroid nodules) after cervical irradiation for HD (50% of cases for Nelson [454]). Surveillance thyroid function tests and cervical ultrasonography thus appear justified for patients treated for HD.

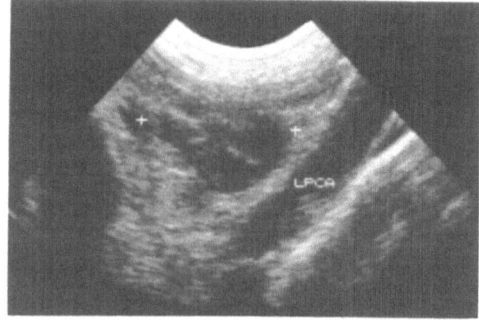

Fig. 4.8. NHL of the thyroid gland. (Transverse scan: 23 mm between the *two crosses*). *LPCA*, left primary carotid artery

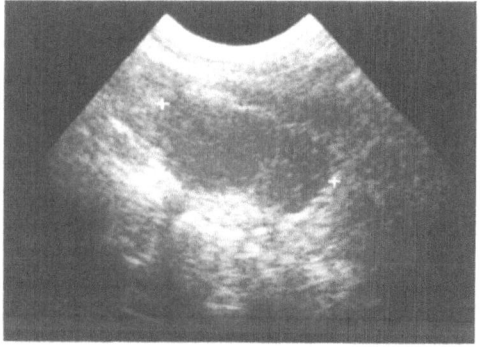

Fig. 4.9. NHL of the thyroid gland. (Sagittal scan; 26 mm between the *two crosses*)

4.4 Salivary Glands

Lymphomas of the salivary glands represent only 0.55% of all primary lymphomas and 4.7% of all extranodal forms [212]; a mere 102 cases were reported between 1948 and 1977 [398]. Salivary gland involvement is much more frequent in NHL than in HD [464], but accounts for only 4% of all lymphomatous masses of the neck [403]. The parotid gland is the site of predilection; the submandibular gland is the site of less than 10% of all primary salivary gland lymphomas [464]. While lymphomas account for 2.8% of all cancers of the parotid gland, the majority of these cases actually concern intraparotid lymph nodes. True primary parotid lymphomas are thus even rarer [563].

As for thyroid gland lymphomas, histiocytic forms predominate. An association between NHL of the parotid gland and benign lymphoepithelial lesions has also been suggested [464]. On a clinical level, women aged 60 or over are affected most often. More or less extensive swelling is common. Well-demarcated swelling can suggest a favorable prognosis, whereas infiltrative-appearing lesions may suggest malignancy from the outset, whether or not there is any associated facial paralysis. The prognosis for primary lymphomas of the salivary glands is slightly less favorable than for other cancers of this site: 67% survival at 5 years and 21% at 10 years [212].

Radiological investigations do not demonstrate any specific sialographic appearances [225].

More recently, three sonographic patterns have been defined [78]:

Localized nodular disease manifesting as strongly hypoechoic, well-limited homogeneous nodules. This pattern suggests a benign mixed lesion, and is a possible source of false-negatives of malignancy for ultrasonography of parotid tumors (Fig. 4.10).

Small multinodular lesions generally corresponding to intraparotid lymph nodes, which readily suggest a lymphomatous etiology, especially when concomitant cervical nodes are also visualized (Fig. 4.11).

Diffuse infiltrating lesions which, like clinical examination, suggest a malignant process. Ultrasound cannot determine the exact depth of extension, however, owing to the superior projection of the mandibular ramus (Fig. 4.12).

Examination must always be completed by exploration of the nodal regions of the neck.

CT is indicated in pretherapy work-ups to determine the depth of extension of diffuse infiltrating lesions and, in particular, to detect any spread toward the pharynx or any bone involvement. Injection of contrast material allows evaluation of the relationships between the tumor and neighboring vessels and detection of any adenopathies [81, 238]. For focal or multiple nodular lesions, however, CT does not appear to provide any additional data to those provided by ultrasound.

4.5 Cervical Adenopathies

The frequency of nodal involvement in NHL varies from 52% to 76% of patients, depending on the series and country of origin [28, 212, 403, 437]. When nodal lesions predominate, the frequency with respect to other cervicofacial manifestations has been evaluated at 8%–49% [93, 403]. This disparity is probably due to the differences in patient recruitment between hematological and surgical services. Cervical node manifestations constitute the only clinical form of cervicofacial HD, owing to the extreme rarity of extranodal cervicofacial HD sites [187].

Clinical examination generally suffices for the detection and diagnosis of cervical adenopathies. Moreover, the therapeutic strategy does not depend on determination of the number of

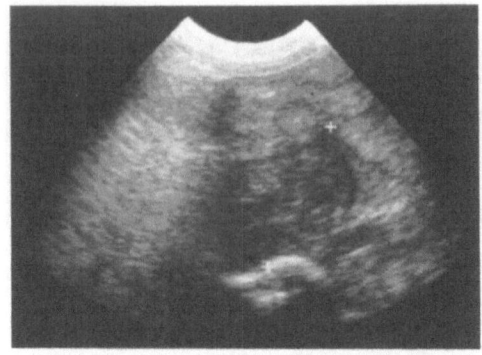

Fig. 4.10. NHL of the parotid gland: 24-mm-diameter nodular lesion (between the *two crosses*), which is less echogenic than the uninvolved parenchyma. (Transverse scan)

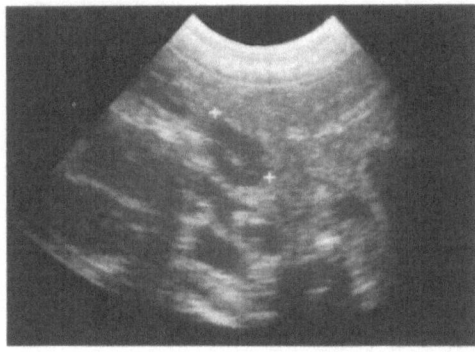

Fig. 4.11. NHL of the parotid gland: diffuse multinodular disease corresponding to intraglandular nodes. (Transverse scan: 11 mm between the *two crosses*)

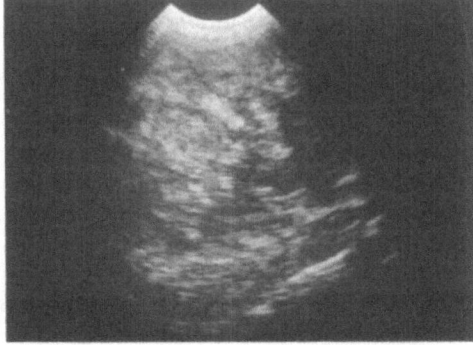

Fig. 4.12. Primary NHL of the parotid gland: infiltrative pattern

nodes involved, in contrast to nodal metastases of head and neck cancers, for which precise anatomical data are essential [80, 408, 409]. Nevertheless, ultrasonography is a valuable adjunct for exploration of lymphomas affecting the cervical nodes. Real-time sonography with a high-frequency transducer (at least 7 MHz) is a rapid, noninvasive procedure suitable for serial use; it can be performed during the same session as ultrasonography of the abdomen and other superficial node regions (axillary, supraclavicular, and inguinal regions). Ultrasonography is more sensitive than clinical examination for the detection of enlarged cervical nodes, both during initial staging and searches for disease recurrence [80] (Figs. 4.13–4.15).

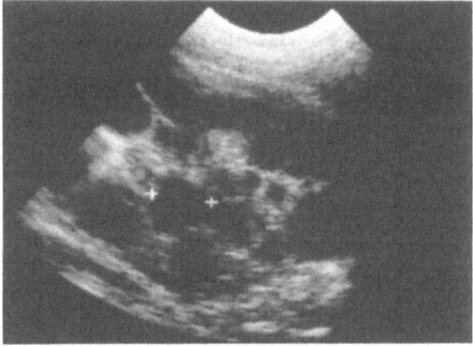

Fig. 4.13. Multiple cervical adenopathies, spinal chain. (Sagittal scan: 10 mm between the *two crosses*)

Cervical adenopathies are generally solid and strongly hypoechoic. In certain instances, and particularly in NHL, nodes can appear to contain fluid. Hypoechoic patterns are more frequent in HD than in NHL, whereas fluidlike images are more common in NHL. The sonographic patterns reflect nodal architecture: on histology sections, NHL nodes are homogeneous, and thus without any interfaces, whereas the more heterogeneous HD nodes give rise to the intranodal interfaces demonstrated on sonograms.

Real-time examinations with high-frequency transducers permit detection of cervical nodes with a transverse diameter of 5 mm. The efficacy of examination varies with the thickness of the patient's neck, since adipose tissue ensures good structural differentiation. Even when nodal masses are very large, they are rarely accompanied by venous thrombosis, in contrast to metastatic nodes.

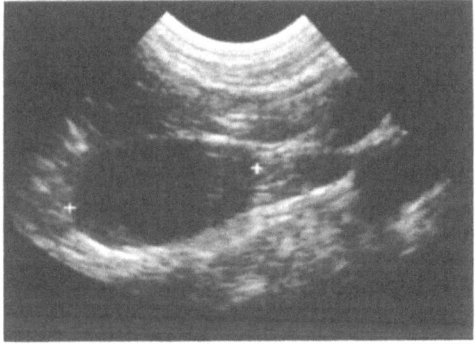

Fig. 4.14. Large lymphadenopathy (28 mm between the *two crosses*)

Ultrasonography of the cervical region has a dual role in cases of lymphomatous nodal disease:

During initial staging work-ups, both the number and precise location of peripheral (and especially cervical) nodes can be defined; the surgeon can be given a diagram indicating lesion sites and diameters. The indications for cervical ultrasonography as a surveillance procedure to evaluate response to treatment can be extended to cover a wide range of patients, or restricted to specific categories. Systematic examinations can be performed at 3 and 6 months, with additional sonograms being obtained at regular in-

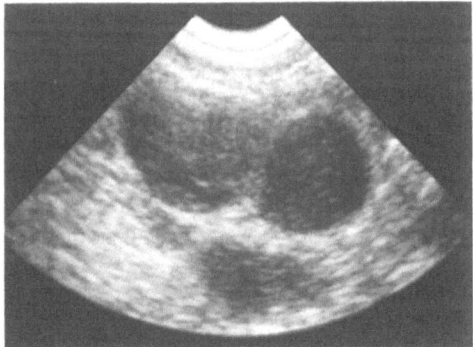

Fig. 4.15. Hodgkin nodes; note the increased echogenicity with respect to NHL nodes

tervals regardless of response to treatment. Another approach consists in performing ultrasound studies at longer intervals, but only for patients difficult to examine clinically, either because they have a thick neck or because irradiation of the cervical region has caused skin thickening. A third, much more restrictive strategy limits cervical ultrasonography to cases in which clinical findings after chemotherapy or radiotherapy are normal, the aim being to confirm the efficacy of treatment.

Whether applied on a wide scale or restricted to the obtention of punctual data as a function of clinical findings, ultrasonography of the cervical region should be incorporated into follow-up protocols for lymphomas.

4.6 Larynx

Laryngeal lymphomas are rare, accounting for only 0.13% of all NHL [161]. Until 1979, only 50 cases had been published [15, 161, 166, 467, 644]. Four clinical forms have been described: isolated involvement, lesions with cervical adenopathies, lesions with distant involvement (retroperitoneal nodes), and laryngeal involvement during generalized disease. Clinical examination reveals a soft, submucosal mass, generally in the supraglottic region, extending to an arytenoid cartilage. The vocal cords and the subglottic areas are rarely involved. The prognosis is good for focal lesions (Figs. 4.16 and 4.17).

4.7 Ear

Lymphomas of the ear are very rare, occurring as polypoid lesions in the external auditory canal. Middle-ear involvement occurs essentially with bulky lymphomas of the nasopharynx [550].

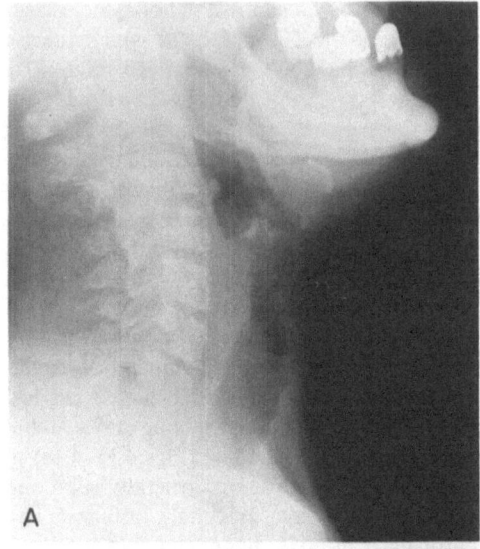

A

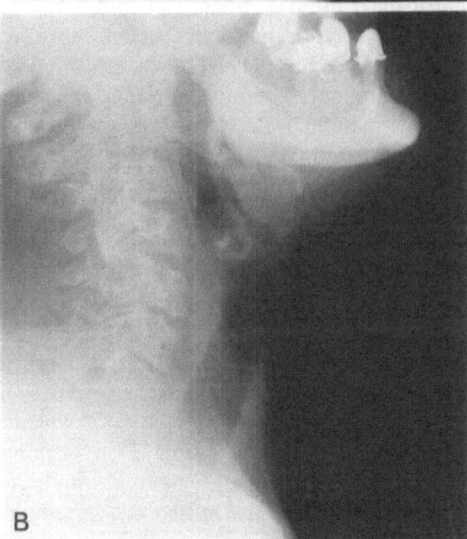

B

Fig. 4.16 A, B. NHL of the larynx. **A** Before and **B** 2 months after irradiation: disappearance of the anterior nodular lesions on the lateral views during phonation

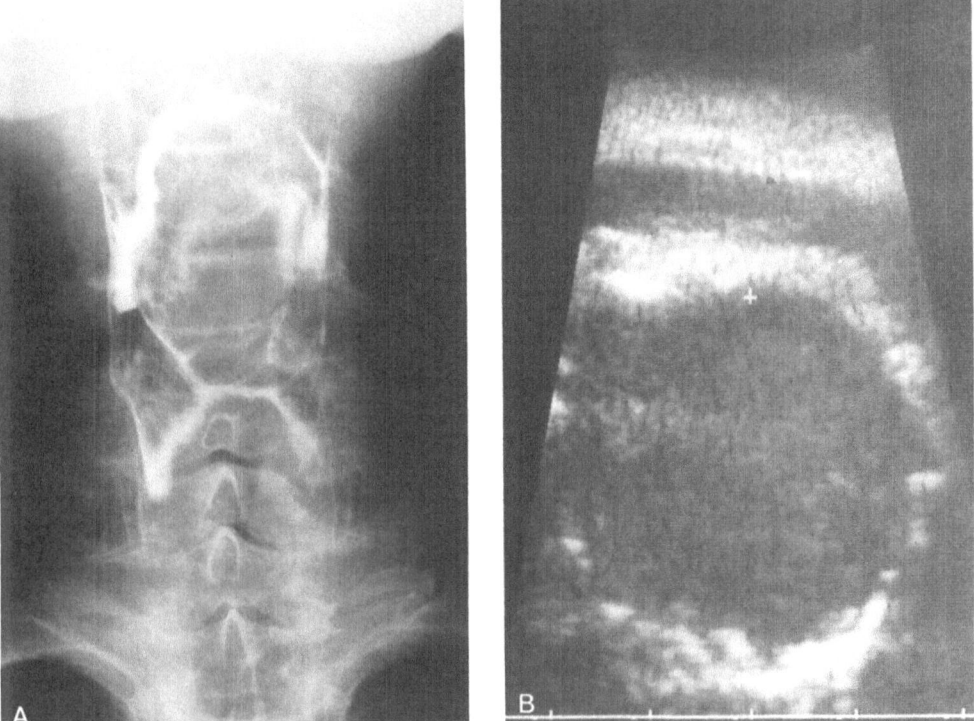

Fig. 4.17 A, B. NHL of the larynx. **A** Laryngography and **B** ultrasound (30 mm between the *two crosses*)

5 Lymphomas of the Thorax

J. FRIJA, M. KATZ, AND M. LAVAL-JEANTET

5.1 Hodgkin's Disease

Chest radiography is of prime importance in all stages of Hodgkin's disease (HD). It can detect HD in asymptomatic individuals; it is essential for initial disease staging; it allows evaluation of response to treatment; and it is indispensable for patient follow-up, since the thorax can be the site of disease recurrence detectable only by radiography. HD commonly affects the mediastinal lymph nodes and the thymus, and more rarely, the trachea, bronchi, heart, and esophagus. The lungs, pleura, and chest wall can also be involved. The frequency of involvement of individual intrathoracic sites varies for initial HD and relapses.

5.1.1 Strategy

5.1.1.1 Radiological Examination

The principal radiological examination of the thorax consists in anteroposterior and lateral chest radiographs. While analysis of radiographs at the onset of HD often allows easy detection of disease in a mediastinal site, diagnosis based solely on subtle contour changes can prove more difficult. Plain chest radiographs judged normal or equivocal are always supplemented by mediastinal tomograms. When radiographs demonstrate a pathologic mediastinum, mediastinal tomograms are of no additional value, since the mediastinum will be included in the radiation field regardless, and tomographic confirmation of lesions obvious on standard films will not alter patient management. By contrast, whole-lung tomography is useful for detecting pulmonary lesions (Fig. 5.1), especially in the presence of hilar nodes. For Kaplan [330], hilar nodes can be precursors of pulmonary involvement.

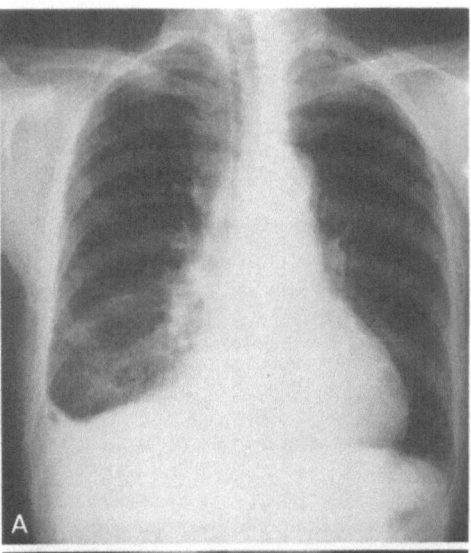
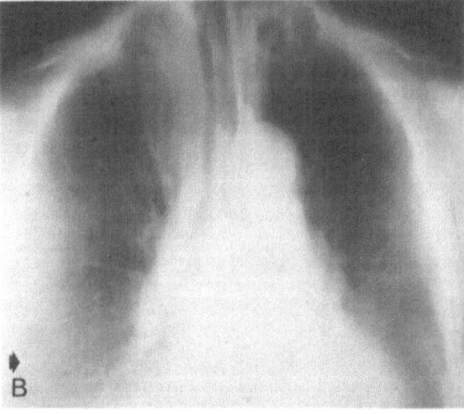

Fig. 5.1. A HD revealed by an interstitial syndrome and right laterotracheal adenopathies. **B** The peripheral pulmonary nodule *(arrow)* was extremely hard to discern on standard films, but was demonstrated by tomography

This theory was corroborated by Castellino [112], who found additional disease sites by lung tomography in 21.4% of 243 untreated patients with HD or non-Hodgkin's lymphoma (NHL). These results had important consequences, since planned treatments were adjusted for 3.3% of the patients and disease staging was corrected for 1.2%; lesions suspected from standard films were confirmed for another 2.1%. Overall, 6.6% of these patients benefited considerably from tomography. Whole-lung tomography is more useful for HD than for NHL. When the mediastinum appears normal on conventional films, it is advisable to obtain confirmation, as the area can then be spared the effects of radiotherapy. Anteroposterior and lateral mediastinal films are advisable in such cases to detect any nodal involvement not visible on standard films.

During the course of treatment of HD, anteroposterior and lateral chest radiographs are indispensable to assess the efficacy of treatment and optimize the target volume for irradiation (Fig. 5.2).

Once initial therapy has been completed, anteroposterior and lateral chest radiographs, along with clinical, biological, and lymphographic findings, permit evaluation of whether the patient has achieved remission.

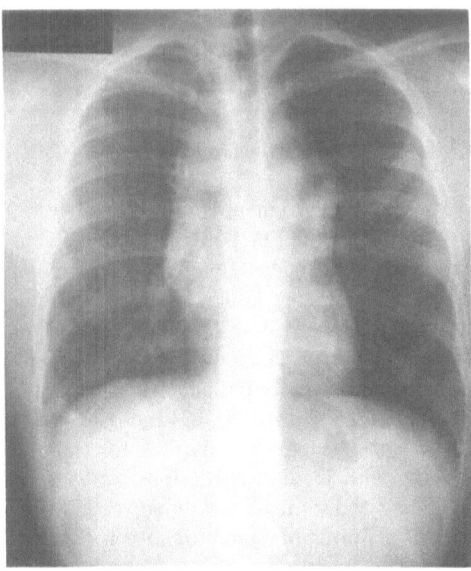

Fig. 5.2. Stage III HD: anterosuperior mass involving the prevascular chain

Correct interpretation of *surveillance films* requires thorough comparison. Since mediastinal irradiation induces juxtamediastinal pulmonary fibrosis, detection of a relapse occasionally depends on the discovery of a minimal change. Thirty-five percent of relapses are solely radiological [112], occurring equally in supra- and subdiaphragmatic sites [327].

5.1.1.2 Computed Tomography

Computed tomography (CT) of the thorax will undoubtedly gradually replace all the existing indications for conventional thoracic tomography (Fig. 5.3). In a retrospective study of 11 patients with HD and 5 with NHL, Kantor [327] analyzed the findings of 21 CT examinations. During initial work-ups, CT confirmed the presence of adenopathies suspected on standard radiographs and mediastinal tomograms in one of five instances. On five occasions, CT proved useful for adapting the fields for mantle irradiation. After completion of irradiation, CT confirmed disease recurrence in one patient and was employed to define the target volume for the boost dose. In another case, CT demonstrated a residual cystic mass; in another it provided no additional information. After chemotherapy and before radiotherapy, CT was responsible for enlargement of the initially planned radiation field for two of four patients. In three cases, CT was of no particular utility. CT thus had therapeutic implications for 11 of these 16 patients investigated by a total of 21 CT studies.

Rostock reported an influence of CT on treatment in 9 of 15 cases (60%) [537]. In three cases, CT demonstrated chest wall invasion, which prompted enlargement of the radiation field. In three other cases, CT was the only modality to reveal pericardial involvement. In still another case, CT revealed nodes lying along the spine and behind the diaphragm, and, in the last two cases, it modified patient staging. These results concur with the work of Pilepitch [501], who reported a modification of radiotherapy fields for 9 of 15 patients. Our experience with CT agrees with the findings of Kantor [327]. Like this author, we have been prevented from compiling a list of indications for thoracic CT, owing to intensive use of our equipment. Never-

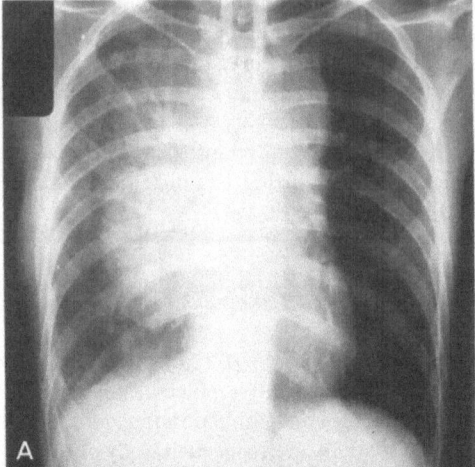
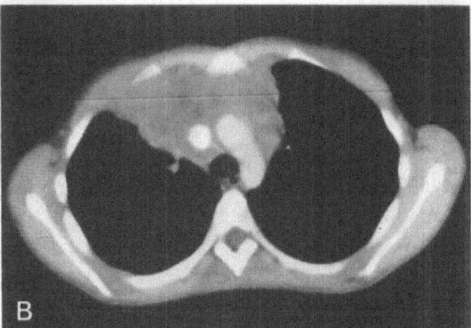
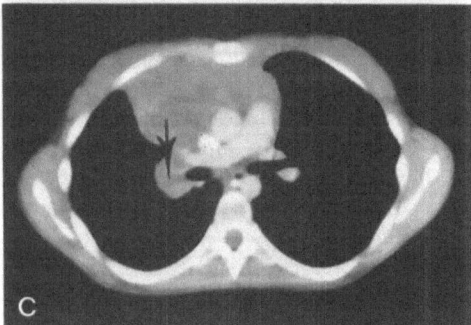

Fig. 5.3 A–C. HD revealed by a solitary thoracic site.
A The Hodgkin lesion has invaded the mediastinum and the vessels. **B** Note the right anterior subpleural involvement and **C** a right hilar adenopathy *(arrow)*

theless, since we feel that CT is superior to conventional radiography for thoracic studies, the range of conditions which indicate it should be increased. For Rostock [537], the purposes served by CT include:

- Evaluation of the extent of disease during initial staging
- Optimization of radiotherapy fields
- Confirmation of complete remission following treatment
- Detection after therapy of a possible residual cystic mass in a wide mediastinum [332]
- Assistance in the difficult analysis of an irradiated mediastinum during the course of HD
- Detection of recurrent disease in the chest wall
- Guidance of transthoracic fine-needle biopsy

5.1.2 Mediastinum

Often asymptomatic, initial involvement of the mediastinum can in rare instances cause a superior vena cava syndrome, or recurrent nerve or phrenic nerve paralysis. Between 50% and 70% of HD patients present with mediastinal lesions from the outset [201, 218, 582]. While 20%–30% of patients have mixed cellularity, 60%–80% have nodular sclerosing HD. Lymphocyte depletion HD is rarely the cause of mediastinal lesions.

5.1.2.1 Prognostic Value and Incidence

Mediastinal involvement is often considered a prognostic factor. For patients treated by radiotherapy, North [469] noted a 5-year survival rate of 88% for stage I and II patients with mediastinal involvement, vs 98% for those without such involvement. There was no significant difference in survival for patients with stage III of the disease (75% vs 78%), but the relapse-free survival at 5 years was only 66% for stage III patients with mediastinal lesions, vs 78% for patients without mediastinal involvement. Fuller [218] reported that the prognosis for stage II patients is actually better when the mediastinum is affected. However, North [469], Mauch [425], and Velentjas [634] have all underscored the poorer prognosis when mediastinal lesions occur in a "large" mediastinum as opposed to a "small" pathologic mediastinum, i.e., in a mediastinum over 7.5 cm wide [469], greater than one-third of the width of the thorax [366, 425], or more than 100 cm^2 [634]. The relapse rate in patients with a wide mediastinum is higher, particularly in the lungs and mediastinum, and nodular sclerosing HD is the predominant histological type. Hilar adenopathies do not influence the relapse rate.

Any of the mediastinal nodes can be affected by HD. Site frequencies vary for initial disease and relapses. In the series of Filly [201], 67% of patients with initial HD had intrathoracic involvement, and 90% of sites were in the superior mediastinum (anterior mediastinum, and paratracheal and/or suprabronchial nodes). Involvement confined to a single lymph node group occurred in only 15% of cases, most often in the superior mediastinum. Solitary involvement of the posterior mediastinal nodes or paracardiac nodes was never observed. The anterior mediastinum was involved in 46% of patients, the suprabronchial nodes in 45%, the paratracheal nodes in 40%, and the hilar nodes in 22%. Subcarinal disease was observed in 12% of cases, but this frequency was probably underestimated, since these nodes are hard to detect. The internal mammary nodes were affected in 7% of cases, the posterior mediastinum in 5%, and the paracardiac nodes in 2%.

5.1.2.2 Radiological and CT Appearances

Any of the nodal chains can be affected. The left and right prevascular chains are often involved, either alone or in association with the thymus. Although it is usually impossible to distinguish the respective roles of nodal disease and thymic lesions in an anterior-superior mediastinal pathology, this relative lack of accuracy has no consequences for therapy. Involvement of this type is thus best referred to as an "anterior-superior mediastinal mass" [333] (Fig. 5.2). CT facilitates analysis of such masses by demonstrating asymmetrical, irregular widening of the superior mediastinum (Fig. 5.4). On lateral views, the retrosternal space is filled in ; the anterior mediastinal line of junction is displaced on tomograms. Occasionally, the lim-

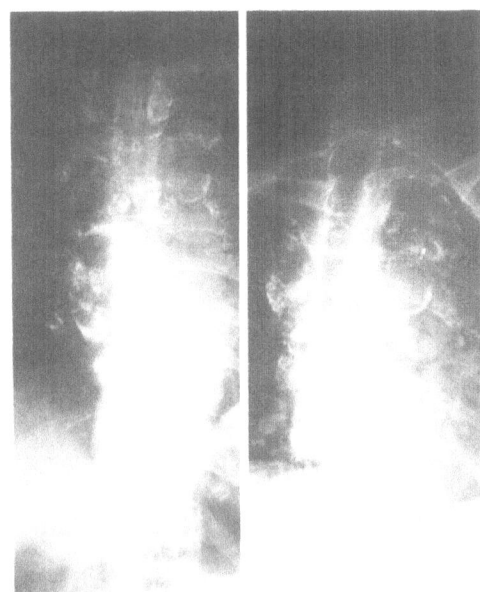

Fig. 5.4. Bulky adenopathies opacified by lymphography in a patient with stage III HD

its are almost vertical, creating a "chimney" image (Fig. 5.5). On the right side of the mediastinum, a second vertical or irregular line is often visible in addition to the azygos vein shadow. On the left side, the supra-aortic region appears enlarged, extending beyond the aortic knob. Below the aortic knob and above the pulmonary artery, where the pleural reflections are normally concave or at most straight, the aortopulmonary window is filled in. A reflection that becomes convex is abnormal, and in a lymphomatous context indicates nodal involvement (Figs. 5.5 and 5.6). Anterior mediastinal masses are occasionally bulky, in which case they can erode the posterior cortical aspect of the sternum. Although visible on lateral radiographs and tomograms, such lesions are far better analyzed by CT.

Whereas anterior mediastinal masses do not extend beyond the upper aspect of the clavicles (Felson's cervicothoracic sign [198]), paratracheal adenopathies can extend higher (Figs. 5.7 and 5.8). On the right, these nodes displace the superior vena cava and the right innominate venous trunk outward; on the left, they lie between the trachea and the aortic arch. When large, they can also extend beyond the vessels

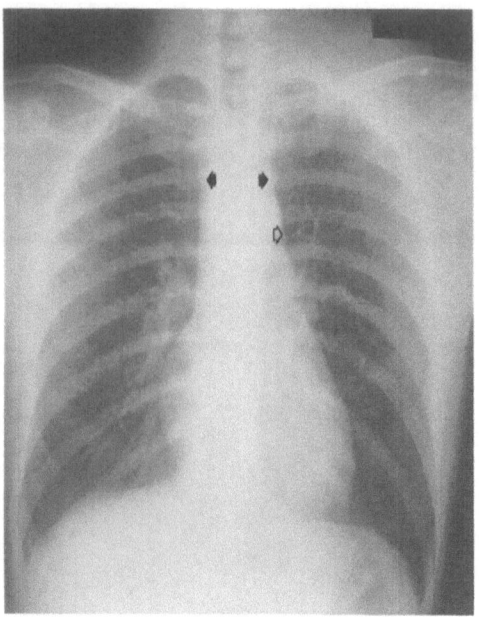

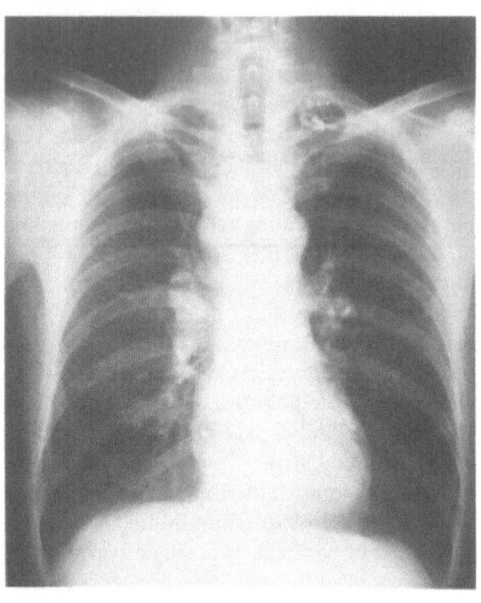

Fig. 5.5. HD with extensive mediastinal involvement *(black arrows)*. A node can be seen in the aortopulmonary window *(white arrow)*

Fig. 5.7. Stage III HD: laterotracheal and right hilar adenopathies. Note the pathologic left supraclavicular node with filling defects opacified by lymphography

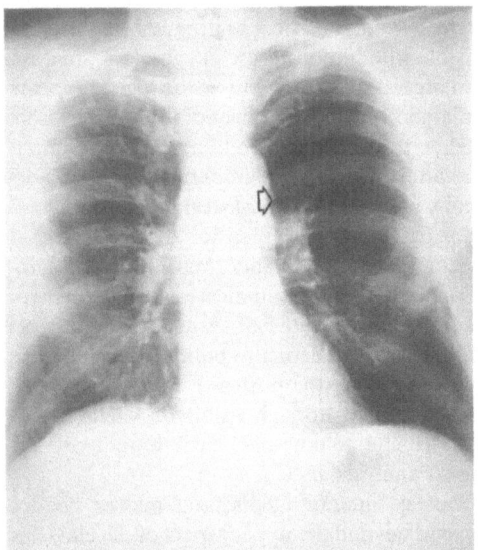

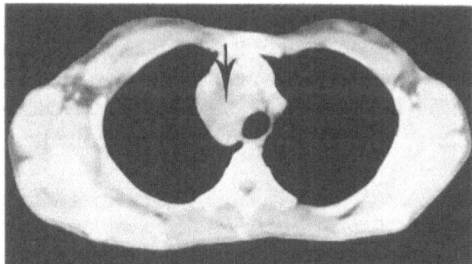

Fig. 5.8. HD revealed by a solitary right laterotracheal mass *(arrow)*. Diagnosis was provided by thoracotomy

Fig. 5.6. NHL. Note the abnormality of the aortopulmonary window *(white arrow)*, which is convex

arising from the aortic arch on the left. The azygos node, the lowest of the right paratracheal nodes, lies in the angle formed by the trachea and the right primary bronchus. Easy to distinguish when large, the azygos node can prove hard to detect when small. Care must be taken to distinguish this node from an arch of the normal azygos vein, whose caliber changes when the patient is examined in the supine position or after a Valsalva maneuver [103].

The subcarinal nodes are difficult to visualize, even on tomograms [51]. On anteroposterior views they displace the azygoesophageal recess to the right. Occasionally, they enlarge the carinal angle. On lateral views (Fig. 5.9), the subcarinal nodes straddle the clear space between the end of the trachea and the origin of the primary bronchi.

The hilar nodes are also frequently hard to see on standard films; in certain instances, they are demonstrated only on tomograms (Figs. 5.3, 5.7, and 5.9). No vessels converge toward these rounded opacities, which are clearly distinguishable from vascular structures.

Involvement of the posterior mediastinal nodes (paraesophageal, para-aortic, paravertebral) causes displacement of the pleural reflections. CT (Fig. 5.10) analyzes these nodes remarkably well, as it does the paracardiac nodes, which can easily be mistaken for pleuropericardial fat shadows on standard films [195] (Fig. 5.11). Comparison of films is especially helpful in these circumstances. Accurate localization of the posterior mediastinal nodes by CT facilitates the delimitation of radiation fields [312].

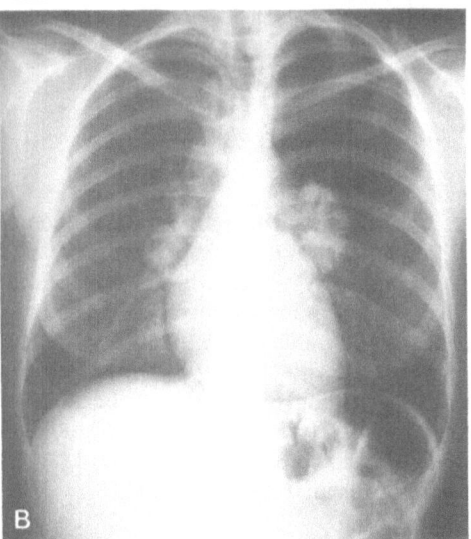

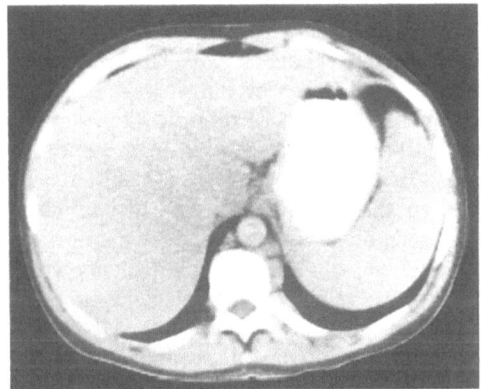

Fig. 5.10. Adenopathies in the posterior inframediastinal space, forming a paravertebral fusiform mass

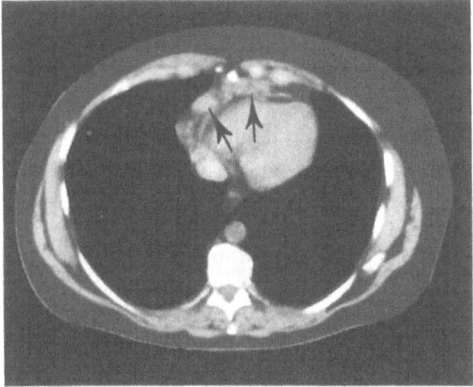

Fig. 5.9 A, B. Stage III HD. Right laterotracheal, bilateral hilar, and subcarinal adenopathies *(arrow)*. These findings are also suggestive of sarcoidosis

Fig. 5.11. Recurrent HD with pericardiac nodes *(arrows)* not visible on the standard films

The internal mammary nodes are visualized on lateral views as an undulating contour immediately behind the sternum. Large nodes can be demonstrated as ill-defined juxtamediastinal opacities on anteroposterior views (Fig. 5.12).

5.1.2.3 Recurrent Disease

The radiological appearances of recurrent disease are the same as those of initial manifestations. For Castellino [112], however, relapses are more frequent in nonirradiated territories (79%). Young [673], on the contrary, reported that the highest incidences of relapse occur in previously involved sites alone (71%) and in associations of previously involved and previously healthy sites (21%). For him, only 8% of relapses occur solely in a previously uninvolved area. Of the 21 patients with an intrathoracic relapse studied by Costello [143], 12 had a nodal relapse, and 9 who originally had superior mediastinal disease relapsed in the same region. Two patients relapsed in the hilum, even though the hila were previously unaffected. One recurrence corresponded to an apical cardiac adenopathy. Of the nine patients with a mediastinal relapse, seven had concomitant recurrence in another thoracic site. Mediastinal adenopathies do not necessarily accompany pulmonary recurrence; the association is frequent for Peckham [490], but rare for Costello [143], for whom seven out of ten pulmonary relapses occurred without mediastinal adenopathies. While detection of obvious recurrences involves no problems, relapses are often masked by the sequelae of mediastinal irradiation. Comparison of chest surveillance films following radiotherapy is essential to detect any contour changes. Nodes lying close to the cardiac apex, simulating a pericardial fat shadow, are invaded almost exclusively by recurrent disease. The delay in their detection emphasized frequently in the literature often stems from failure to compare chest films [143, 195, 331]. When doubts persist despite comparative analysis, CT is indicated to accurately distinguish the mediastinum from the juxtamediastinal radiation-injured lung [382, 480].

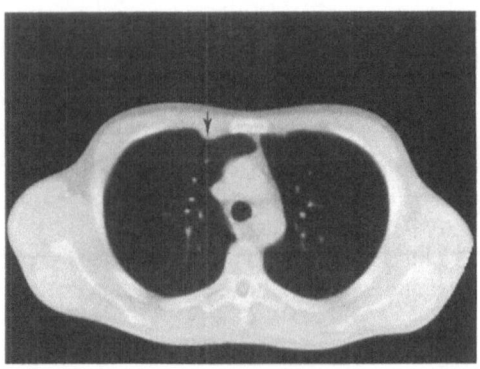

Fig. 5.12. Subphrenic, left supraclavicular stage III HD. The chest radiograph is normal, but CT demonstrates an internal mammary node *(arrow)*

5.1.2.4 Residual Mediastinal Masses

Despite effective radiotherapy, certain patients retain a wide, although stable, mediastinum over several film series. One possible cause is a residual mediastinal mass (Fig. 5.13). While these masses may no longer contain any Reed-Sternberg cells [177], both cystic degeneration (1.6% of HD cases [332]) and calcification of cyst walls [332] are possible. Thymic cysts account for most of these residual masses [332, 562]. In addition to its excellent investigation of such masses [32], CT is useful for guidance of transthoracic fine-needle biopsies. The latter, however, are diagnostic only when positive.

5.1.2.5 Nodal Calcification

Nodal calcification (Fig. 5.14) occurs in 1.6%-2.4% of patients following radiotherapy [72]. Spontaneous nodal calcification is exceptional, and only one case has been published [462]. Calcification has been observed 1-14 years after irradiation with 10-60 Gy [668]. There are not usually any specific characteristics [278], although eggshell calcification has been reported [158, 668]. The site of predilection is the anterior mediastinum [245, 278], followed by the hilar nodes [158, 662].

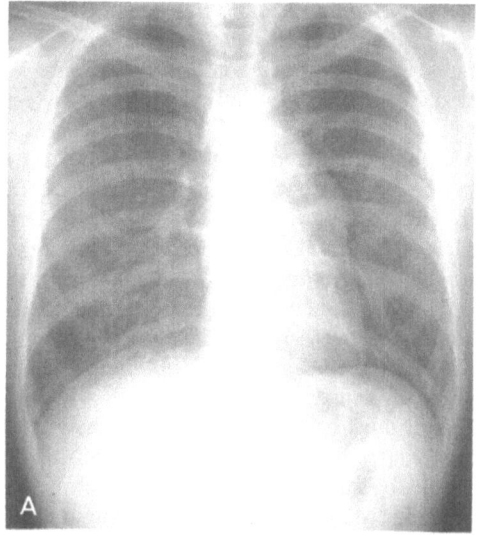
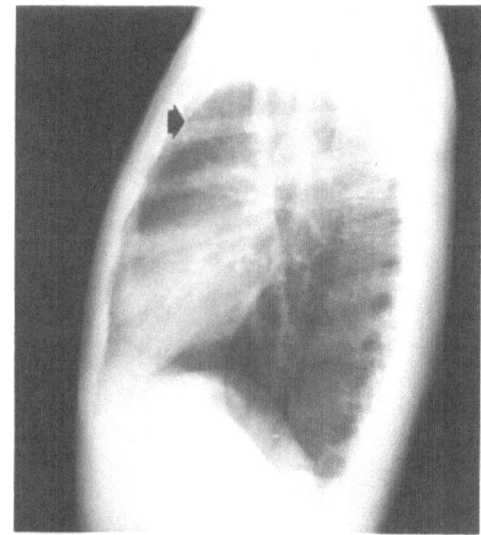
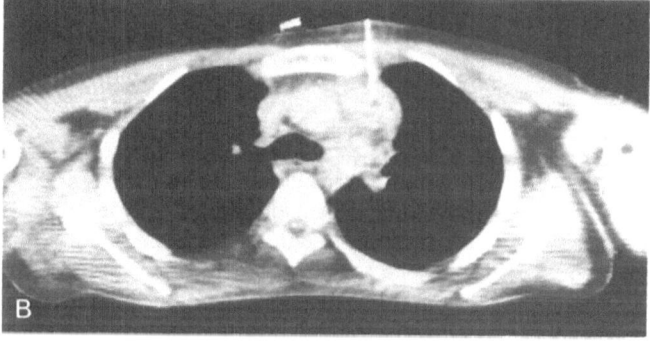

Fig.5.13 A, B. Stage II HD. A Residual thymic mass; B CT-guided puncture and evacuation of acellular fluid

Fig.5.14 *(upper right)*. Calcified retrosternal nodal mass *(arrow)* that appeared after radiotherapy

5.1.2.6 The Irradiated Mediastinum

Owing to the frequency of mediastinal involvement by HD, analysis of surveillance films often concerns an irradiated mediastinum (Fig. 5.15). The development of visible sequelae of radiotherapy depends on personal factors: a given radiation dose will cause juxtamediastinal pulmonary fibrosis in some patients, but not in others.

Radiation pneumonitis appears after 30–35 Gy, and almost always occurs above 40 Gy [383]. Chemotherapy, and corticosteroids in particular [115], appear to lower the dose threshold for pulmonary radiation injuries. Chemotherapy followed by irradiation with 40 Gy leads to radiation pneumonitis in approximately 8 weeks.

In our experience, radiation pneumonitis is often visible on CT scans as soon as radiotherapy is completed, and in all cases 1 month later, when chemotherapy is administered as the initial treatment modality. Radiation pneumonitis nearly always progresses to postirradiation fibrosis, which stabilizes in 9–12 months [387]. Modifications in the pulmonary parenchyma occur solely within the radiation field. Radiation-induced lung injuries are thus clearly demarcated, with margins corresponding to the limits of the radiotherapy fields. CT accurately evidences such lesions.

The intensity of radiation pneumonitis is variable during the early stages. In certain cases,

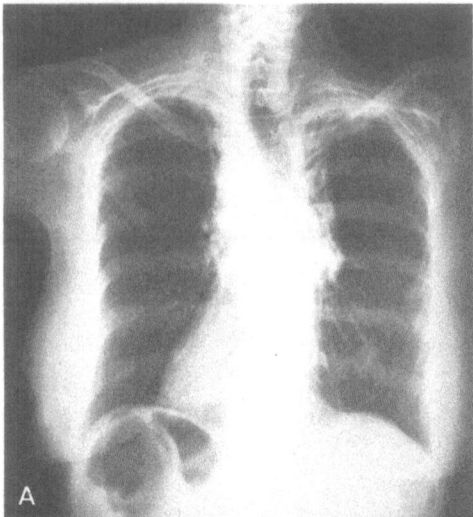

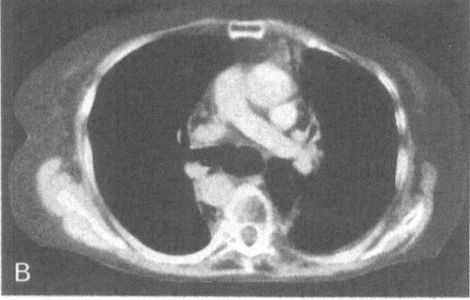

Fig.5.15 A, B. Postirradiation patterns. **A** The mediastinum is hard to analyze on the standard film. **B** CT accurately distinguishes the juxtamediastinal pulmonary radiation fibrosis from the mediastinal elements

only a juxtamediastinal shadow is visible, and the pulmonary vessels are poorly delimited. In other cases the reaction is severe, producing a juxtamediastinal pulmonary opacity containing an air bronchogram. The more severe the radiation pneumonitis, the more pronounced the postirradiation fibrotic sequelae. Radiation pneumonitis rarely regresses. The severity of postirradiation pulmonary fibrosis is also variable, and it can even occur in the absence of any previously visible radiation pneumonitis [384]. The mediastinal contours are blurred; the apical vessels become more vertical and are pulled toward the mediastinum. The minor fissure and the hila may be elevated; occasionally only the hila are elevated [262]. Contraction can occur, modifying the distribution of the vessels

in the remaining healthy parenchyma. Elevation of the diaphragm can take place in severe cases. Radiation pneumonitis can be accompanied by pleural effusion, which generally regresses. A spontaneous [379] or recurrent [624] pneumothorax is a rare finding. Chemotherapy can favor radiation-induced pulmonary lesions [498, 499]. Resumption of chemotherapy – with, namely, doxorubicin hydrochloride (Adriamycin) [399] – after radiotherapy not complicated by radiation pneumonitis can provoke radiation lesions not visible before chemotherapy.

Although there are several differential diagnoses for a juxtamediastinal radiation-injured lung, it must be remembered that radiation fibrosis is radiologically stable; complications should be suspected when modifications are detected. Mantle irradiation including the supraclavicular fossa leads to fibrosis in the clavicular region. Tuberculosis can be entertained as a possibility. Postirradiation pulmonary fibrosis occasionally suggests lymphangitis carcinomatosa, although this last pathology generally occurs in a different clinical context and is usually more visible at the lung periphery (Kerley's lines). The major difficulty is detection of recurrent disease in an irradiated site or at the edge of a radiation field; the best solution is to search for radiological modifications by comparing films.

5.1.2.7 Heart

Primary lymphoma of the heart is very rare [130, 525], although lymphomatous cardiac lesions are not uncommon findings at autopsy [480]. The incidence of cardiac involvement is higher in NHL (approximately 25%), and in particular in mycosis fungoides (33%), than in HD (10%). Any region of the heart can be affected, but involvement of the valves is infrequent. Tumors are occasionally noted on surgical specimens in the form of small nodules; large lesions are rare. Cardiac sites of HD often consist in microscopic invasion, with no visible tumor. Radiological and clinical signs are both rare, although symptoms are somewhat more common in HD.

In those patients who present with cardiomegaly, the most common diagnostic problem is differentiation from radiation-induced pericarditis. The frequency of radiation pericarditis in

HD varies from 6.6% to 30% of patients after 40 Gy [542, 594]; the incidence is even higher when the mediastinum is initially very wide [362]. Using CT, we detected pericardial thickening in 4 (31%) of 13 patients 4 months after completion of a radiotherapy course. Radiographically demonstrable cardiomegaly is often asymptomatic, and can precede clinical manifestations; it can appear 4–12 months [383 or even 10 years [19] after irradiation. Ultrasound cardiography [416] and CT should allow more accurate detection of pericardiac reactions in the future.

Radiotherapy appears to increase the risk of coronary-related deaths [56]; coronography [615] can detect coronary stenosis and the atheromatous buildup which appears accelerated in such situations. Abnormalities of this type are not mandatory, however. Yahalom [669], for example, reported myocardial infarction in a 19-year-old woman 27 months after 44-Gy mantle irradiation, despite normal coronary studies. Chemotherapy, and especially doxorubicin hydrochloride with its recognized cardiac toxicity, potentiates the harmful effects of irradiation of the heart.

5.1.2.8 Esophagus

HD of the esophagus, a rare entity, is discussed in Chap. 7.

Acute esophagitis, occasionally caused by *Candida* [598], can occur following irradiation with over 30 Gy [383]. The acute symptoms resolve with symptomatic treatment. There are usually no radiological signs, although irregularities are occasionally noted in the mucosal folds. Phillips [499] found no esophageal lesions in a series of 300 patients after a certain interval had passed since radiotherapy.

5.1.2.9 Great Vessels

Compression of the superior vena cava and/or the innominate venous trunks is rare in HD, and only slightly more frequent in NHL [388]. Post-irradiation lesions of the great vessels usually produce no clinical manifestations, except when radiation fibrosis of an innominate venous trunk occurs within an irradiated mass.

5.1.2.10 Trachea and Bronchi

Only 13 cases of tracheal lymphomas have been published, reflecting the rarity of these lesions [404]. Lymphomas differ from other tracheal neoplasms in that they are usually disseminated; focal lesions are rare.

Endobronchial sites of lymphoma are very rare, but can occur during relapse. Fifteen cases have been reported (7 of HD, 6 of NHL, 2 of "malignant lymphoma"). These nodular lesions are occasionally polypoid. Bronchial obstruction is possible [30], and investigation of an endobronchial lesion may even result in the diagnosis of HD. Thirteen cases were collected by Harper, who added four of his own [265]. Single or multilobar ventilation abnormalities are frequent consequences. Pleural effusion can accompany atelectasis, and hilar nodes are frequent (9 of the 13 cases compiled by Harper).

Bronchodigestive fistulas can develop during the course of lymphomas of the esophagus (as in epidermoid carcinoma), or the stomach (in cases of an associated diaphragmatic hernia, a subphrenic abscess, an infiltrating tumor surrounding the stomach and extending to the thorax, or trauma [592]).

5.1.3 Lungs

5.1.3.1 Initial Manifestations

Initial involvement of the lung by HD is rare, and accounted for only 11.6% of the cases in the series of Filly [201] and 12% in the series of Aghai [5]. Lesions of this type are rarely solitary; when a pulmonary lymphomatous site is detected on a chest radiography (Fig. 5.16), other sites are often discovered on tomograms [118]. Initial pulmonary lesions are bilateral in nearly half of all cases [18, 201]. When the pulmonary lesion is located near the mediastinum and can be included in the radiation field, it does not alter the prognosis [490]. When the pleural reflection on a mediastinal or hilar nodal mass is blurred rather than sharply defined, extension of nodal disease to the lungs can be suspected. Lesions distal to the mediastinum correspond to stage IV disease, which has a less favorable prognosis [18]. Initial pulmonary le-

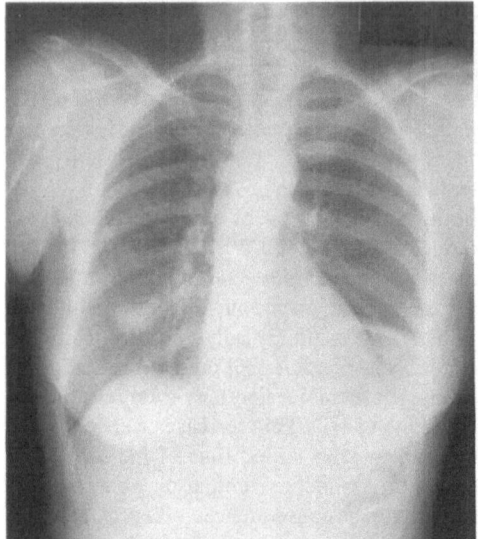

Fig. 5.16. Early pulmonary site of HD

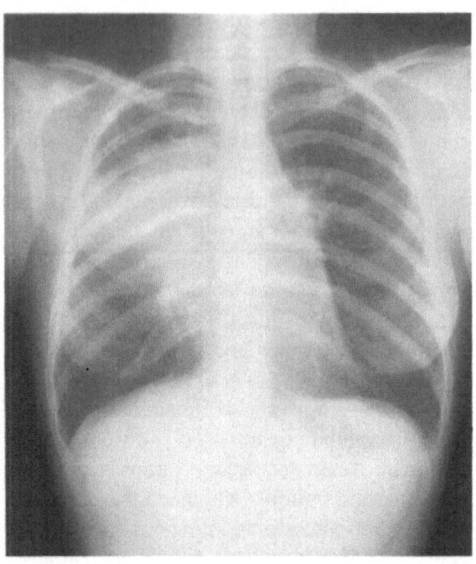

Fig. 5.17. HD with tumoral infiltration simulating atelectasis, limited on the bottom by the minor fissure. Note the right hilar adenopathies

sions are almost always [18] accompanied by mediastinal adenopathies, and especially hilar nodes [201], although solitary pulmonary involvement has been reported [255, 338, 438, 490]. Nodular sclerosing HD accounted for 48% of cases for Peckham [490] and 85% for Andrieu [18]. In this last series, 80% of the patients presented with general symptoms, and all had biological signs of progressive disease. In contrast to initial HD lesions, pulmonary relapses are not invariably associated with mediastinal adenopathies.

Stohlberg [595] has described three modes of diffusion of HD in the lung: (a) pulmonary infiltration along the vessels and bronchi ("bronchovascular infiltration"), which occasionally become obstructed; (b) subpleural diffusion (although the pleura may appear thickened, peripheral pulmonary nodules are present); and (c) massive pneumonic infiltration, possibly with cavitation. Pulmonary lesions are demonstrated radiologically as small or large nodules with sharply or ill-defined margins. These nodules can be cavitary, in which case they may be thick-walled with irregular margins and contain a fluid level [576]. The differential diagnosis for thin-walled nodules is tuberculosis: only response to treatment can differentiate the two

[576]. Bronchi with thickened walls and poorly defined vessels may be visualized between nodules and the hila (Fig. 5.10), but such findings are not pathognomonic [33]: the cause can be lymphatic stasis above a mediastinal mass rather than true cellular infiltration [595].

In certain cases, poorly delimited infiltrates are present. Infiltrates tend to coalesce, producing homogeneous shadows of recognizable segmental or lobar distribtution containing an air bronchogram (Fig. 5.17) as the result of alveolar collapse or alveolar filling by malignant cells. During treatment, these opacities can cavitate [490]. In rare instances, impaired ventilation secondary to endobronchial infiltration produces atelectasis, and it is difficult to distinguish the ventilation disorder from actual cellular infiltration. Ventilation impairment as the result of endobronchial spread is rare [250]. Infrequently, nodal compression of a bronchus causes atelectasis. Miliary lesions are exceptional [490, 539]. The interstitial syndromes noted on occasion resolve rapidly with treatment, and are often caused by lymphatic engorgement secondary to compression by a mediastinal mass.

5.1.3.2 Recurrent Disease

Pulmonary relapses are most frequent in nodular sclerosing HD [490], and the lungs in general are frequently involved by recurrent disease (12% of cases for Young [673]). The characteristics of recurrent disease (Fig. 5.18) are the same as those of initial lesions, except that the incidence of pulmonary sites is higher (10 out of 21 intrathoracic relapses in the series of Costello [143], 12 out of 31 in the series of Castellino [112]), and association with mediastinal nodes is less common (three out of ten in the series of Costello and Mauch [143]). For Kaplan [330], hilar nodes present at the outset are the precursors of disease in pulmonary sites. He thus advocates preventive irradiation of the lung (15 Gy) when hilar nodes are detected, even in the absence of discernible pulmonary lesions. Pulmonary calcifications are rare, occurring exclusively after radiotherapy [598]. Pulmonary alveolar proteinosis has been reported during progressive HD [102].

Large pulmonary nodules occasionally persist following chemotherapy, but these sterilized, stable residual masses contain no Reed-Sternberg cells. Intrathoracic (pulmonary, mediastinal, parietal) residual masses are most common in nodular sclerosing HD [373].

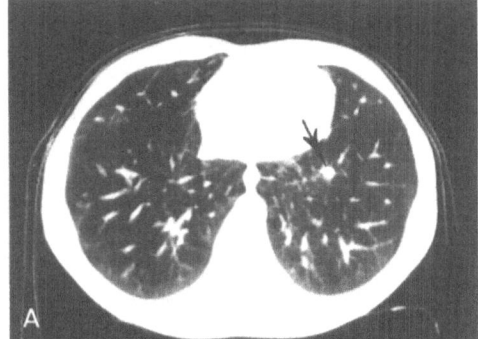
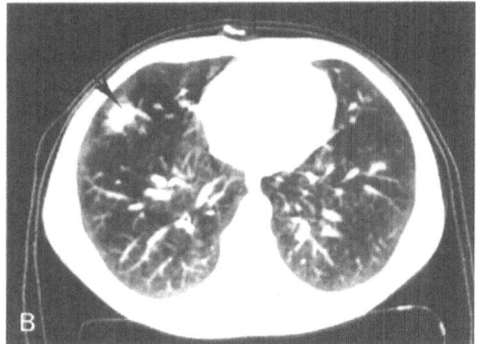

Fig. 5.18 A, B. Two CT scans demonstrating pulmonary relapse of HD in the form of two nodules (arrows) which were difficult to detect on the standard film

5.1.4 Pleura, Chest Wall, and Diaphragm

5.1.4.1 Pleura and Chest Wall

Pleural effusion (Figs. 5.19–5.21) usually, although not invariably, carries a poor prognosis in lymphomas. While HD can be confined to the pleura, it is often impossible to differentiate between pleural effusion secondary to a purely pleural site and mechanical obstruction in lymphatic drainage pathways [647]. Pleural effusions frequently regress as mediastinal nodes decrease in size in response to treatment. Cytologic study of pleural fluid frequently yields negative results, and even the presence of lymphomatous cells in a pleural effusion does not automatically correspond to a pleural site of lymphoma [647]. An effusion of a chylous nature does not modify the prognosis. Stohlberg [595] has described pleural lesions as thick plaques which are not necessarily accompa-

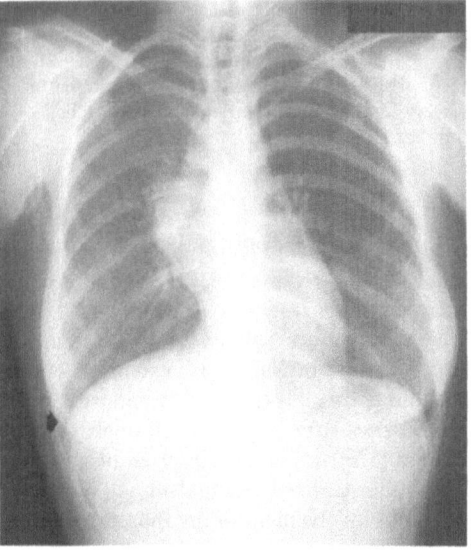

Fig. 5.19. Stage II HD. Right pleural effusion of mechanical origin (arrow), which disappeared with regression of the right hilar, right laterotracheal, and subcarinal nodes (hypoplasia of the right first rib)

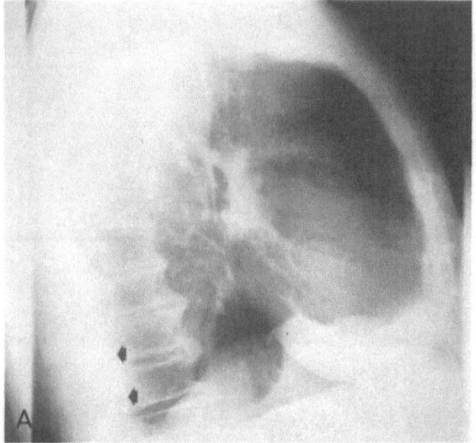

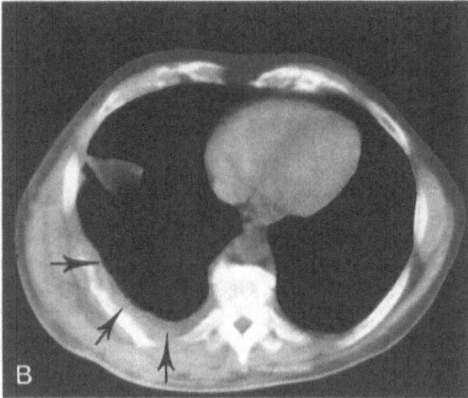

Fig. 5.20 A, B. Relapse of HD. **A** Subpleural invasion by HD is very difficult to see on the lateral film
(arrows). **B** CT scan through the right eighth rib,
which is partially destroyed. Note the subpleural invasion *(arrows)* and enlargement of the chest wall
muscles

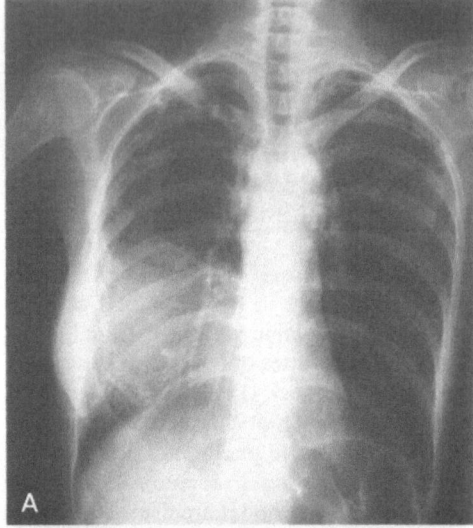

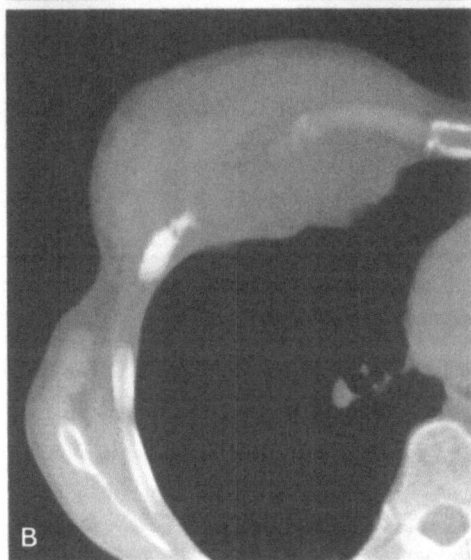

Fig. 5.21 A, B. Bulky HD recurrence invading the
breast and destroying the chest wall (lysis of the
fourth and fifth ribs)

nied by effusion. Pleural plaques habitually
occur during relapses of HD and NHL. CT
analyzes these lesions particularly well [576],
whether they are solitary or associated with
costal lesions, in which case extension outside
the thoracic wall is possible. Response to treatment varies from regression through cyst formation [576], to persistence of an occasionally
large but sterilized residual mass [373]. Concomitant involvement of the thoracic wall and
diaphragm is not rare, and is easily demonstrated by CT.

5.1.4.2 Diaphragm

HD of the diaphragm is rare (2%) [333] and difficult to detect, although Stohlberg [595] reported 7 cases in a series of 50 autopsies. Diaphragmatic lesions are generally seen in HD involving the anterosuperior mediastinum, and especially in cases of postradiation mediastinal fibrosis. Differentiation between involvement of
the upper and lower parts of the diaphragm is

important for both physiopathological and prognostic reasons: subdiaphragmatic involvement appears more severe in superior sites than in intrathoracic sites [618]. Upward displacement of a cupula, whether or not it is associated with fasciculation, is sufficient cause to suspect diaphragmatic involvement even though it may be masked by a suprajacent pleural effusion. Demonstration of diaphragmatic thickening requires lateral decubitus films, insufflation of air into the stomach or even pneumoperitoneum [618]. These techniques allow determination of whether the anterior or posterior diaphragm is involved, since the anterior subpleural lymphatics correspond to the thoracic drainage of the internal mammary nodes, whereas the posterior subpleural lymphatics are drained by collector vessels toward the subperitoneal network and the lumboaortic nodes [618]. CT greatly facilitates investigation, especially of the right cupula, which is hard to distinguish from the liver on standard films.

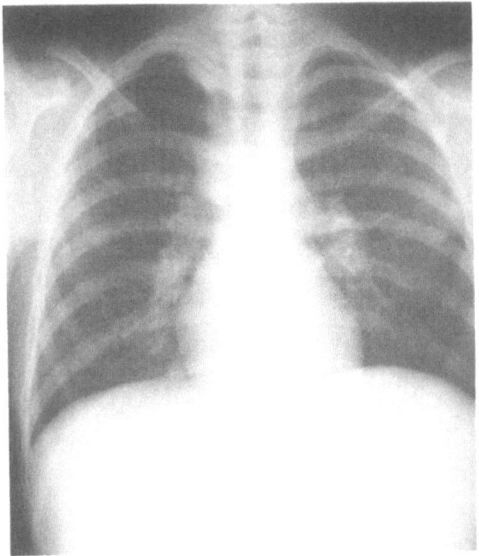

Fig. 5.22. Relapse 3 years after diagnosis of axillary stage I HD in a patient aged 13 years. Bilateral hilar and mediastinal adenopathies

5.1.5 Childhood Hodgkin's Disease

The radiological features of childhood HD (Fig. 5.22) are the same as those of disease in the adult, although the frequencies of specific types of involvement differ. Mandell [410] reported a particularly high incidence (55%) of tracheobronchial compression in a series of 20 cases. Initial intrathoracic sites occur in 62%–64.7% of cases [252, 349, 486], although the incidence is significantly lower in children under 10 years of age (36%) than in adolescents aged 13–16 years (76%) [486]. Nodular sclerosing HD accounts for 70% of cases in adolescents, whereas nodular sclerosis and mixed cellularity each represent 38% in the younger age group [486]. Initial pulmonary involvement is rare in children under 10 (3%), but more common in adolescents (14%). The global incidence is between 13.3% and 14.3% [252, 349]. The association of mediastinal nodes and hilar adenopathies is more common in the younger group (61%) than in the older patients (46%) [486]. Tomograms appear useful only when the mediastinum is pathologic, or when standard anteroposterior and lateral films are suspicious, since they facilitate detection of hilar nodes and pulmonary sites [486].

5.2 Non-Hodgkin's Lymphomas

The symptomatological features of intrathoracic NHL are the same as those of HD. Nevertheless, the intrathoracic site frequencies of NHL differ from those of HD; they also differ according to the type of NHL. Lesions may be suggestive of the diagnosis, or be associated with other clinically diagnostic sites, and, in particular, nodal involvement.

5.2.1 Strategy

During initial work-ups for NHL, anteroposterior and lateral radiographs generally suffice for the evaluation of the extent of disease. Tomograms are of little utility. Castellino [118], for example, reporting on a series of 95 NHL patients investigated by whole-lung tomography, discovered that tomograms corrected the staging and altered previsions for treatment in only one case (1.1%), by revealing a pathology not suspected from standard films.
CT should replace tomography, especially for evaluating the response of tumors to treatment. In certain instances, CT-guided puncture biopsy of residual masses is indicated to detect any

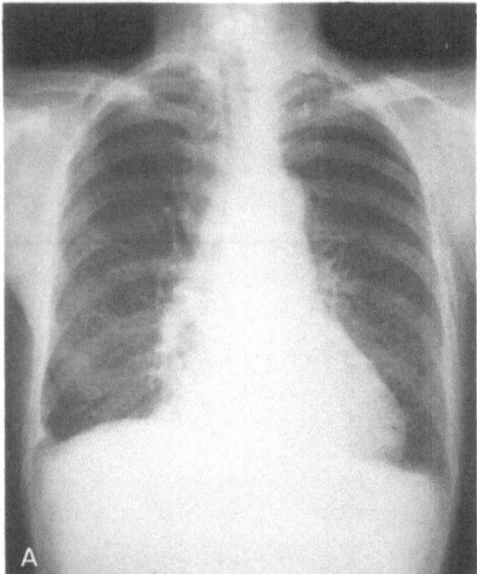

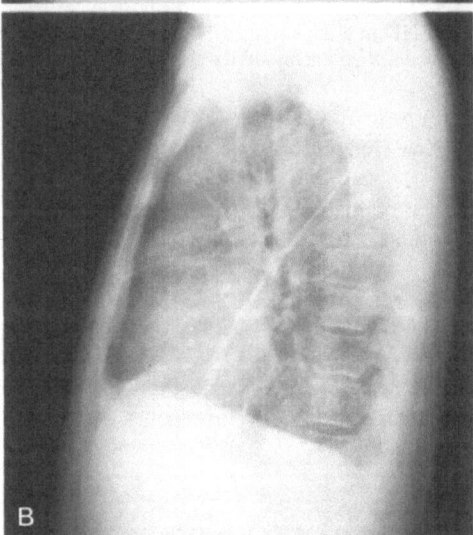

Fig.5.28 A, B. Interstitial syndrome during a nodular lymphoma (**A**). Note the distinct appearance of the thickened fissures on the lateral plain film (**B**)

neoplasms in 3.4% of patients; the autopsy incidence was even higher (6.1%). Likewise, Libshitz [385] observed 23 lung cancers in 2708 cases of lymphomas, whereas only 7 were normally expected.

5.2.2.2 Histological Type

Apart from Filly [201], who reported a high incidence of intrathoracic involvement in 135 patients with NHL (43%), most other series identify thoracic sites as the cause of 18%–22% of all cases of NHL [376, 386].

The frequencies of nodular and diffuse forms are similar. Patchevsky [487] reported mediastinal involvement in 18% of 293 patients: 16% of the 293 had nodular NHL and 20% had diffuse NHL. Forty percent of the mediastinal sites corresponded to nodular NHL, and 60% to diffuse NHL. In his series of 405 cases, Jones [317] noted initial mediastinal and/or hilar involvement in 18% of patients with nodular NHL and in 24% with diffuse NHL. Although the mediastinum was unaffected in this series, lower cervical and/or supraclavicular nodes were present in 40% of the nodular NHL cases, in 20% of the diffuse NHL cases, and in 28% of all lymphomas considered together. Strauss [596], analyzing 499 cases, found left hilar nodal involvement in 17% and right hilar nodal involvement in 19%. No mention was made of mediastinal involvement, but 5.6% of patients had pulmonary sites of NHL, and 8.3% had pleural lesions.

The frequency of thoracic and/or mediastinal involvement varies with the histological type of NHL. For Bennet [41], the incidence of mediastinal involvement is:

- 12% in nodular, poorly differentiated lymphocytic NHL
- 20% in nodular, mixed NHL
- 14% in nodular, histiocytic NHL
- 35% in diffuse, poorly differentiated lymphocytic NHL
- 12% in diffuse, mixed NHL
- 13% in diffuse, histiocytic NHL
- 11% in diffuse, undifferentiated NHL
- 0% in diffuse, well-differentiated lymphocytic NHL

In his study of 112 cases of *histiocytic NHL*, Burgener [84] diagnosed lymphoma on the basis of clinical and/or radiological signs and symptoms in 12 cases (11%). After the disease had progressed for more than 2 years, 56 patients (50%) had thoracic involvement consisting in a mediastinal mass (25%), hilar nodes (17%), pulmonary lesions (20%), pleural involvement (18%), or lymphomatous sites in the chest wall (14%). Nineteen patients had unilateral (2 cases) or bilateral (17 cases) hilar involvement; bilateral nodes were associated with pulmonary and/or mediastinal lesions.

Lymphoblastic lymphomas account for one-third of all childhood lymphomas and 5% of adult lymphomas. Between 50% and 75% of cases involve mediastinal sites [304, 331, 450, 529], but these lesions are rarely solitary. Of the 95 patients studied by Nathwani [451], 42 had mediastinal NHL sites, and 30 of them (75%) were male. Mediastinal involvement is more frequent in patients under 30 years of age than in patients over 30 ($p = 0.001$).

Large mediastinal lesions are most frequently seen in diffuse large-cell NHL [263, 376, 386, 621], during which sclerosis plays an important role, and in lymphoblastic NHL [263]. Seven (6.5%) of the 107 patients with diffuse histiocytic lymphoma studied by Miller et al. [434] had a relatively localized mediastinal mass, but extensive sclerosis. Mediastinal masses can be solitary (6% for Levitt [386]) or associated with other lesions, especially adenopathies (40% of the 30 patients investigated by Harousseau [263]), and sites in the spleen and spine.

Pleural effusions are not uncommon (50% for Harousseau [263]); they are often of mechanical origin, as are pericardiac effusions, which are less frequent. Contiguous pulmonary lesions are common (4 of 30 cases of Harousseau [263]). Trump [621], reporting on 11 patients with a predominant mediastinal mass (10 diffuse large-cell lymphomas, 1 diffuse undifferentiated non-Burkitt's lymphoma), noted hilar nodes in 10 patients, pleural effusion in 8, and a contiguous pulmonary lesion in 5. CT detected pericardiac infiltration in two instances. These histological types are commonly responsible for residual mediastinal masses which remain stable following therapy. Local and/or generalized recurrences progress rapidly [263, 621].

Both mediastinal and pulmonary involvement are rare in *American Burkitt's lymphoma* [677]. In a series of 40 patients, Dunnick [176] observed pleural effusion which was due to a mechanical cause in 9 cases (7 associated with ascites), mediastinal adenopathies in 2 cases, and bilateral mediastinal and hilar nodes in 1 case. Krudy [352] utilized CT to investigate 29 patients, and found 7 who had both an anterior and a posterior mediastinal lesion, each of which was associated with a cervical or abdominal nodal mass. Four of the five patients with a pleural effusion also had ascites.

Foucar [208], studying 47 patients with *diffuse mixed lymphomas*, noted 5 mediastinal lesions (10.6%), 2 pleural lesions, 2 pulmonary lesions, 2 cardiac lesions, and 1 tracheal lesion.

Twenty-two (20%) of the 112 patients with *histiocytic NHL* investigated by Burgener [84] had pulmonary involvement.

Fourteen patients (13%) had an *interstitial infiltrate* varying from reticular to reticulonodular in appearance. Twenty of the patients had *hilar adenopathies* (hilar lesions that fail to respond to therapy progressively enlarge and extend toward the lungs, and complex interstitial and alveolar or even pseudoedematous lesions are then possible). Of the 22 patients, 9 were found to have *pulmonary nodules* (solitary in 2 cases, multiple in the other 7), varying in size from several millimeters to several centimeters. These nodules were well circumscribed in half of the cases, but had blurred contours in the other half. Frank cavitation was never observed. In four of the patients these pulmonary nodules constituted the only intrathoracic sites of involvement; the remaining five patients had associated hilar nodes and/or other disease sites. Two patients had only multiple primary pulmonary nodules. Five of the six patients with mass lesions or consolidation (5%) also had disease in other intrathoracic sites; the last patient no longer had any other lesions when pulmonary involvement was diagnosed. The extent of consolidations varied from subsegments to entire lobes; consolidations were solitary in three instances and multiple in the three others. Twenty (18%) of the 112 patients had pleural involvement (unilateral in 7, bilateral in 13); the pleural plaque constituting the initial manifestation in four cases later progressed to extensive pleural effusion. Pleural effusion was the sole initial manifestation in two cases; in the other cases it was a late occurrence associated with disease in thoracic and/or extra-thoracic sites.

Sixteen patients had thoracic bone lesions: mixed lesions were more common than purely lytic or sclerotic forms. Fifty-two (46%) of the 112 patients in this series had peripheral node involvement. Intrathoracic sites of lymphoma were the third most frequent manifestations leading to diagnosis after nodal and abdominal lesions. In 11% of patients, disease was confined primarily to the thorax.

In a series of 11 patients with *T-cell lymphoma associated with human T-lymphotrophic virus (HTLV)* and characterized by rapidly progressive disease, Bunn [83] observed the rapid appearance of hilar adenopathies (4 of the 11), without mediastinal involvement, and pulmonary lesions in the form of bilateral infiltrates (5 of the 11). The course of the disease, which included cutaneous and peripheral nodal dissemination, was associated with a paraneoplastic syndrome including hypercalcemia, an elevation in alkaline phosphatases, and a normal bone scan with increased uptake reflecting increased bone turnover. Of the 11 patients, 4 had osteolytic lesions.

Mycosis fungoides is a cutaneous T-cell lymphoma, which remains localized in the skin for long periods. The prognosis deteriorates once nodal and/or visceral lesions develop. Pulmonary involvement is a common finding at autopsy, occurring either as microscopic disease or nodules (21 of 32 cases for Rappaport [516]), but is rarely detected during life as it occurs late in the course of the disease. Pulmonary involvement is usually associated with peripheral adenopathies [516] (Fig. 5.29), and is demonstrated radiologically as unilateral or bilateral, solitary or multiple nodules (six times out of ten), poorly defined infiltrates, or interstitial involvement, which is most prevalent at the lung bases [414]. Associated linear atelectasis is possible [660], as are mediastinal and/or hilar adenopathies [516, 660]. Pleural effusion can be an associated or solitary finding, and massive pulmonary infiltration of rapid onset has been reported [300]. Since radiological images are not specific, diagnosis requires cytologic analysis of puncture material or histological examination of biopsy specimens. This is all the more true since pulmonary lesions in these patients

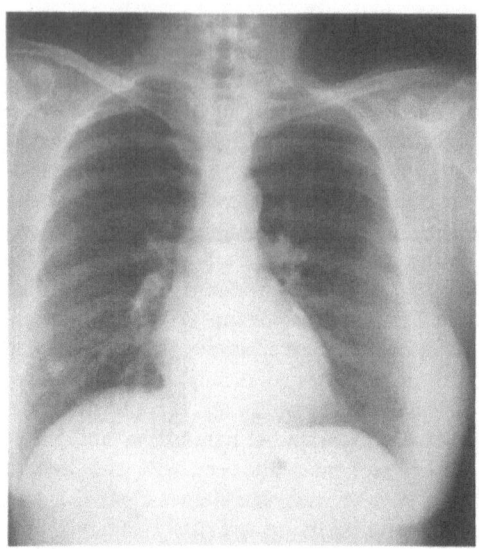

Fig. 5.29. Terminal mycosis fungoides with two nodules in the right lung

are often caused by opportunistic infections, as revealed by autopsies [660].

5.2.3 Primary Lymphoma of the Lung

Primary lymphomas of the lung develop at the expense of the organ's lymphoid structures [415]. Freeman [212] reported 53 pulmonary lesions in his series of 1467 extranodal lymphomas. Based on his literature review of 121 cases, Gebauer [228] cited an average patient age of 52 years. The right lung is affected more frequently (71%) than the left. In view of the incidence of relapses (4%) and metastases (23%), surgery is advisable. The postsurgery survival rate is 54.5% at 2 years and 25.5% at 5 years. Half of all primary pulmonary lymphomas are asymptomatic or accompanied by nonspecific pulmonary signs [294]. Hypertrophic pulmonary osteoarthropathy has been described in connection with one case [40]. Primary lung lymphomas are demonstrated radiographically as a poorly defined homogeneous mass in one or more lobes which can contain an air bronchogram [484]. Masses tend to be located centrally rather than peripherally, and are extrabronchial, extravascular, and extra-alveolar. As the tumor grows within the interalveolar septa, the adjacent lung tissue is compressed. Multi-

ple opacities are rare, and are generally unilateral. Infiltrates are generally surrounded by numerous nodules; micronodules have been reported in relapses [294]. Hugues [294] reported 10 cases of contractile consolidations, 8 instances of associated pleurisy, and 5 cases of cavitation in his literature review of 137 cases.

While involvement of the hilar nodes is possible, the mediastinal nodes are usually unaffected. The radiological findings are often misinterpreted as lung cancer, and the correct diagnosis is provided only by cytopathological analysis, even though primary lung tumors are characterized by a very slow growth rate.

6 Nodal Lymphomas of the Abdomen

J.-N. Bruneton, E. Caramella, and J.-J. Manzino

Modern imaging modalities have greatly contributed to current knowledge about intra-abdominal nodal lymphomas. Since both intra- and retroperitoneal node involvement can be demonstrated by computed tomography (CT) and ultrasonography, it seems legitimate to treat these two sites together in the same chapter, particularly since the older separation between intraperitoneal and retroperitoneal nodal disease was based to a large degree on the limitations of lymphography. This separation now appears unnecessary, especially for non-Hodgkin's lymphomas (NHL), since exploratory procedures for subdiaphragmatic NHL sites have been extensively revised in recent years. By contrast, Hodgkin's disease (HD) has benefited less from recent technological advances.

Retroperitoneal involvement occurs in 49% of all cases of NHL (68% for nodular disease, 25% for diffuse forms) and in 25% of HD cases [236, 237, 260]. The intraperitoneal nodes are involved in 51% of cases of NHL (71% for nodular disease, 27% for diffuse forms) but in only 4% of cases of HD. This diversity in the incidence of nodal involvement between HD and NHL, the diagnostic capabilities of modern imaging techniques, and the histopathological features of lymphomatous non-Hodgkin and Hodgkin nodes, justify adoption of an investigatory approach which takes all of these factors into account. Details of this investigative strategy are discussed following a review of available imaging modalities.

6.1 Imaging Modalities

Plain abdominal radiography, urography, and vascular opacification techniques are reviewed only briefly, as they have been supplanted by newer modalities.

Aside from surveillance films taken after lymphography for follow-up purposes, *plain abdominal radiographs* are of little utility in themselves. Large masses can be detected when they cause displacement of gas-filled intestinal loops. More rarely, after radiotherapy [245, 401], nodal lesions are demonstrated as mottled calcifications or irregularly calcified masses. The unproven explanation of this phenomenon is related to cellular necrosis, which has a high calcium uptake potential.

Cavography and *urography* are no longer employed for intra-abdominal studies. In HD nodal involvement, one or the other of these techniques reveals abnormalities in a third of cases [361].

Arteriography has also been abandoned as a diagnostic procedure. In the past, arteriography occasionally evidenced avascular lesions, but the usual finding was irregular vascularity with nonhomogeneous staining during the capillary phase [374].

In current practice, the four main methods for the exploration of abdominal lymph nodes are lymphography, ultrasonography, CT, and radionuclide studies. The first three techniques are also utilized to guide biopsies for staging purposes and for the evaluation of response to treatment.

6.1.1 Lymphography

Lymphography is the oldest of the currently used diagnostic procedures. A review of the general features of this method as applied to lymphomas is followed by discussion of the different patterns observed, the problem of differential diagnosis, and the overall accuracy of the technique.

Lymphography can accurately examine the iliac and lumbo-aortic chains, but cannot evaluate the celiomesenteric nodal regions. Easy to perform, and even to repeat a second or third time, lymphography allows assessment of the response of retroperitoneal nodes to treatment on surveillance abdominal films (anteroposterior, lateral, two obliques). In two-thirds of cases, however, there is no longer enough residual contrast material 18 months after lymphography to permit satisfactory evaluation [192, 593]. After 2 years, only 12% of patients can still be assessed by plain abdominal radiography [593]. Because of this limitation, and of the frequency and time of occurrence of HD relapses, lymphography must be repeated once initially opacified nodes are no longer visible [328]. Complications are generally rare (less than 1% for Macdonald [397]) when contraindications are respected (especially severe respiratory impairment).

Lymphograms allow study of the anatomical distribution of disease sites as well as the characteristics of individual nodes, such as diameter, margins, and storage pattern [281] (Figs. 6.1 and 6.2). Lymphographic findings for HD are remarkable for their great heterogeneity [21, 554]. Few of the lymph nodes opacified are actually affected, and all of the various radiological patterns are possible, although the different pictures depend on the extent of involvement.

Findings for initial Hodgkin lesions include more or less regular filling defects, moderate enlargement in nodal diameter, and the absence of stasis. Such appearances are common to all inflammatory processes, and are thus nonspecific. By contrast, discovery of a normal-sized node containing a well-delimited filling defect [405] represents one of the main indications for early films, which reveal the circulation abnormalities (occlusion, bypass, increase in number of visible vessels) present in 42% of all cases of retroperitoneal nodal HD [478]. Diagnosis is easier for more diffuse and larger lesions; findings include stasis, nodal enlargement, and large, irregular filling defects with dense zones. Very large lesions can even result in nonopacified nodes [358].

All of the above findings can be observed in HD, especially in nodular sclerosing and mixed cellularity types. Histiocytic NHL can have similar appearances, but without lymphatic stasis.

NHL lymphograms are notable for their homogeneous character: all of the affected nodes have the same appearance and all exhibit the same degree of abnormality. Filling defects are uncommon, and stasis is less frequent than in HD [21, 554]. No pattern specificity exists for subtypes [546, 617], and foamy, granular, and

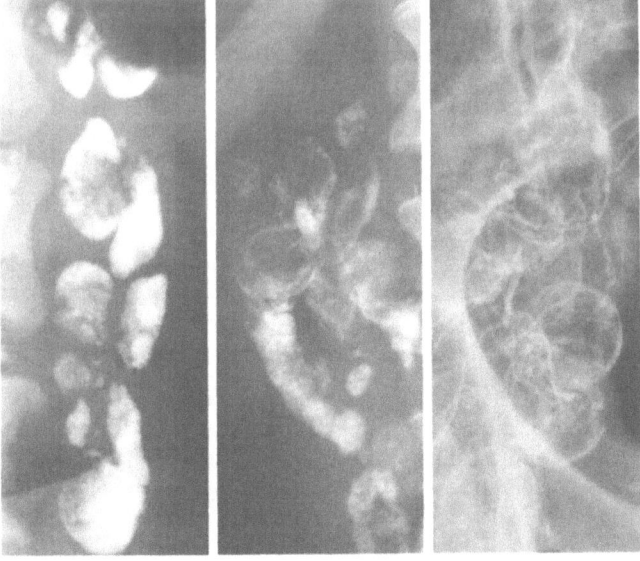

Fig. 6.1. Various filling defects observed in lymphomas. *From right to left:* HD, NHL, AIL (angioimmunoblastic lymphadenopathy)

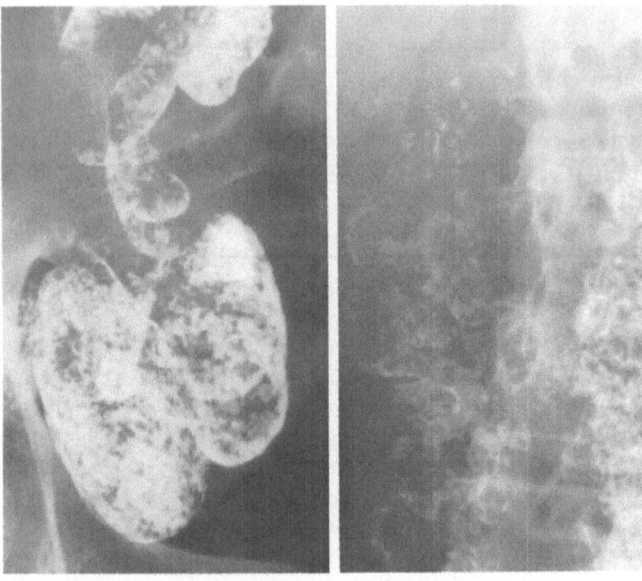

Fig. 6.2. Several types of foaminess

lacy structures have all been described. These lymphographic findings are more particularly associated with poorly and well differentiated lymphocytic and mixed lymphocytic-histiocytic NHL. A similar appearance is possible for a particular form of lymphocyte predominance HD, but the latter is also usually accompanied by filling defects [554].

Angioimmunoblastic lymphoadenopathy (AIL) exhibits a somewhat special pattern, since only the peripheral sinuses are preserved. More often diffuse than localized. AIL is more marked at the iliac level than at the lumbo-aortic level. The typical reticular or lacy pattern has sharp, well-defined margins; granular patterns are less common [76].

For both HD and NHL, the patterns observed after a repeat lymphography are comparable to those seen after initial procedures. Nevertheless, certain particularities warrant mention:

1. Comparison with the initial lymphograms allows detection of relapse [593]: nonopacification of previously opacified nodes, diffuse nodal enlargement with respect to initial diameters, enlargement of a group of lymph nodes, modifications in internal architecture and nodal homogeneity, and node displacement by a nonopacified mass.

2. Local disease recurrence is less frequent after radiotherapy than after chemotherapy. Comparison of first and second procedure lymphograms generally reveals regression in node size, irregular contours, and intranodal filling defects (Fig. 6.3). The most marked changes are seen in those nodes involved by the disease process from the outset [113, 173, 382].

3. Reactive follicular hyperplasia, a source of false-positives observed almost exclusively on repeat lymphographies [111, 114, 173, 485], manifests as diffuse, symmetrical nodal enlargement and increased nodal granulation. This rare phenomenon (less than 10% of second lymphographies) is most frequent in children, and occurs in the absence of any prior chemotherapy or radiotherapy. The etiology of reactive follicular hyperplasia remains unclear, although reaction to the contrast material used during the first procedure has been suggested as a possible mechanism.

In addition to the false-positives caused by reactive follicular hyperplasia, which occurs under particular circumstances, and to the inability of the technique to opacify the celiomesenteric nodes, lymphography involves several other diagnostic problems:

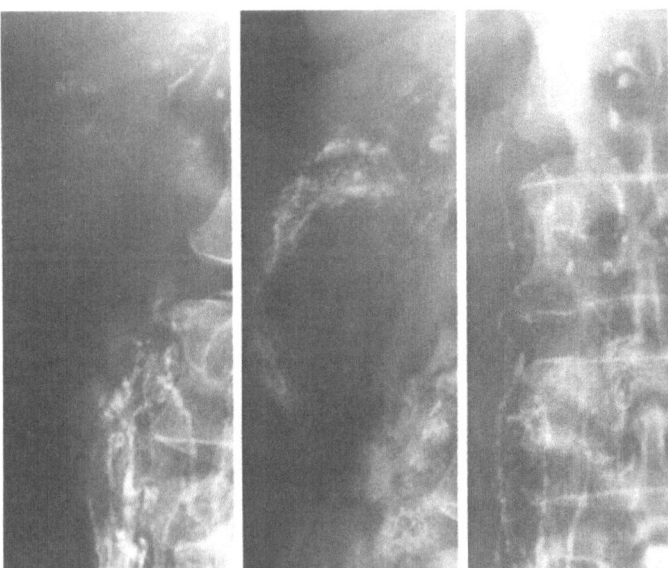

Fig. 6.3. Lymphograms of a patient with HD showing a lumbo-aortic nodal mass; film taken during injection *(center)* and 2 days later. One year after treatment, repeat lymphography *(left-hand film)* revealed a decrease in nodal opacification

Rare instances of false-negatives have been reported for microscopic HD lesions [323]. Etiological diagnosis remains the most common difficulty. Diffuse enlargement and granular patterns, for example, also occur in immunological incompetence (dysglobulinemia, hypogammaglobulinemia), granulomatous disease, and infection [485]. A foamy or lacelike internal architecture is not specific either, since metastatic nodes, especially metastases of testicular, ovarian, and renal cancers [397], can exhibit a similar appearance [119, 120]. Likewise, lymphomatous nodes can appear metastatic [119, 120], as in HD when normal-sized nodes show a filling defect [397].

Despite these diagnostic limitations, lymphography globally remains an excellent technique for lymphomas. The method has a sensitivity of 85%–93% for HD and 87%–89% for NHL [116, 121, 413]; its specificity varies from 92% to 98% for HD and is on average 86% for NHL [121, 413]. The overall accuracy of lymphography is thus between 69% and 97% for HD [29, 114, 116, 121, 144, 235, 405, 413, 551] and between 83% and 86% for NHL [121, 413].

6.1.2 Ultrasonography

Owing to the many possible sites of involvement of the iliac, lumbo-aortic, and intraperitoneal nodes, ultrasound imaging is limited from the start by certain inherent technological factors. Exploration of the subpancreatic region, for example, is often prevented by the presence of bowel gas. Ultrasonography is considered technically impractical in 12%–14.5% of cases [405]. Neumann [458] has even declared it insufficient for satisfactory analysis of all of the abdominal and pelvic regions. Whereas the iliac regions are very often difficult or impossible to analyze, the celiomesenteric region is probably the zone for which ultrasonography is the most useful imaging technique (Fig. 6.4). Lymphomatous nodes exhibit a strongly hypoechoic structure. Owing to their homogeneity (particularly in NHL), which sets up few or no interfaces, they can appear cystlike [77, 284, 335, 442, 626] (Figs. 6.3–6.7). Postradiotherapy sonograms can detect both regression in node size and structural changes such as the appearance of more echogenic zones of fibrous origin (Fig. 6.8).

Taking into account those cases for which ultrasonography is insufficient or technically im-

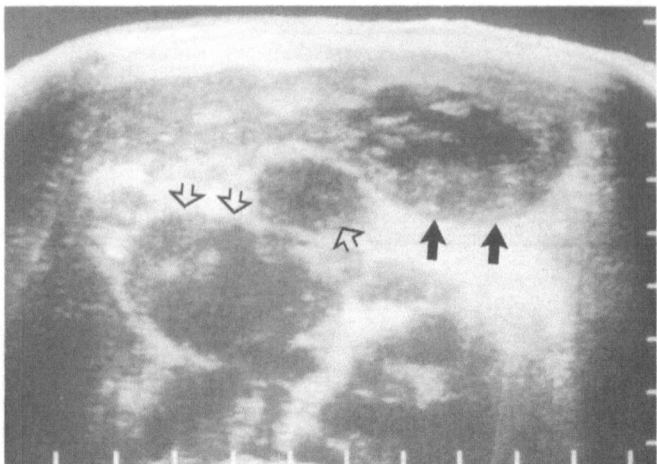

Fig. 6.4. Lymphomatous celiac nodes *(white arrows)* and those associated with hepatic involvement *(black arrows).* (Transverse scan)

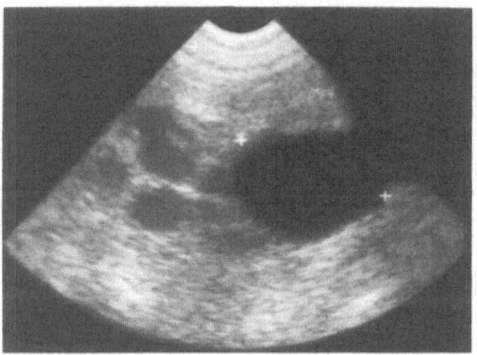

Fig. 6.5. Mesenteric NHL site: fluidlike sonographic appearance. (Transverse scan: 46 mm between the *two crosses*)

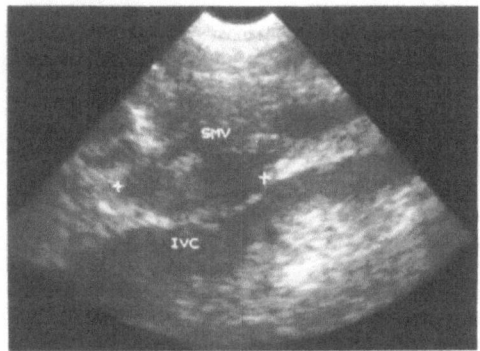

Fig. 6.7. Retroperitoneal HD nodes (Sagittal scan: 45 mm between the *two crosses*). *IVC,* inferior vena cava; *SMV,* superior mesenteric vein

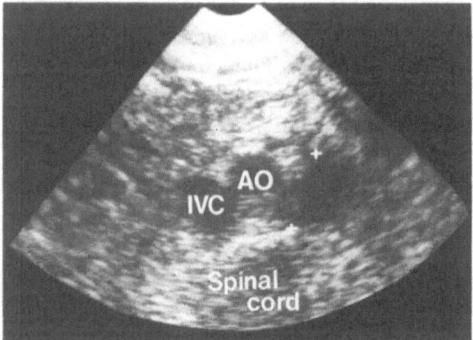

Fig. 6.6. Left latero-aortic lymphomatous nodes. (Transverse scan: 27 mm between the *two crosses*). *IVC,* inferior vena cava; *AO,* aorta

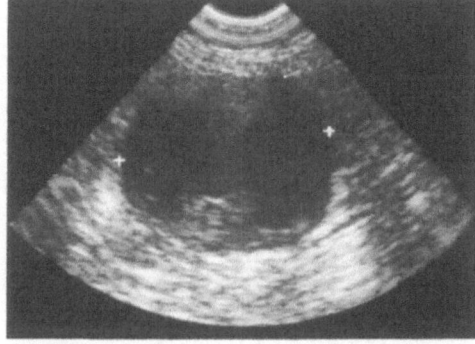

Fig. 6.8. Distal fibrosis of a treated lymphomatous mesenteric NHL node. (Sagittal scan: 58 mm between the *two crosses*)

practical, this technique has a sensitivity of 87.5% [24, 66, 346]. For Brascho [66], the overall accuracy of ultrasonography is 97% when associated with gallium-67 studies. The main indications for ultrasonography are investigation of the celiomesenteric region in thin patients and guidance of puncture biopsies [405].

6.1.3 Computed Tomography

Technological advances have considerably increased the role of CT during the past few years. Whereas in 1977 [8] the indications for CT were restricted to advanced clinical stages, recent prospective studies have emphasized the preponderant role of CT, especially for NHL (Figs. 6.9–6.16). Current technology permits examinations of such high quality that CT findings may be used to modify prior clinical staging. CT is responsible for modifying the clinical stage in 16.2% of HD cases [49], vs 8.2% for lymphography and approximately 35% for laparotomy [49, 551]. In NHL, CT modifies the clinical stage in 14.2% of cases [457].

Subdiaphragmatic nodes are considered abnormal when their transverse diameter exceeds 1.5 cm; nodes under 1 cm are deemed normal.

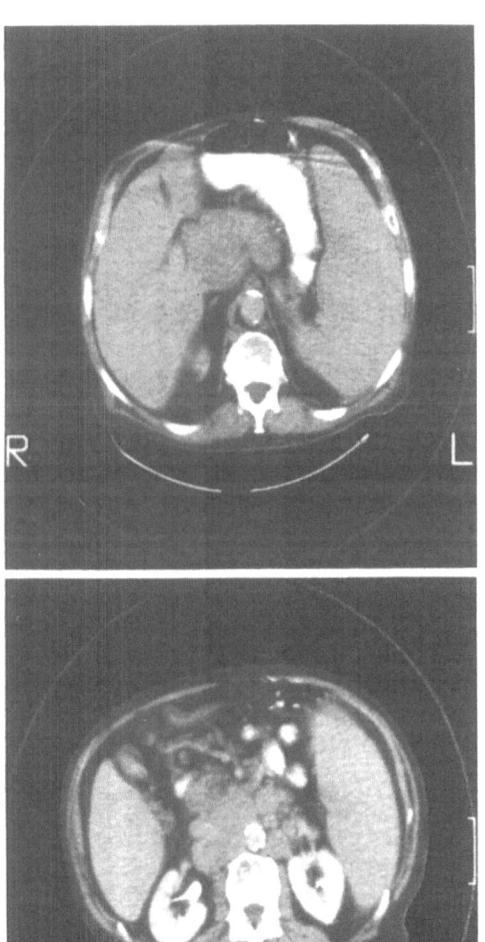

Fig. 6.9. Subdiaphragmatic NHL nodes

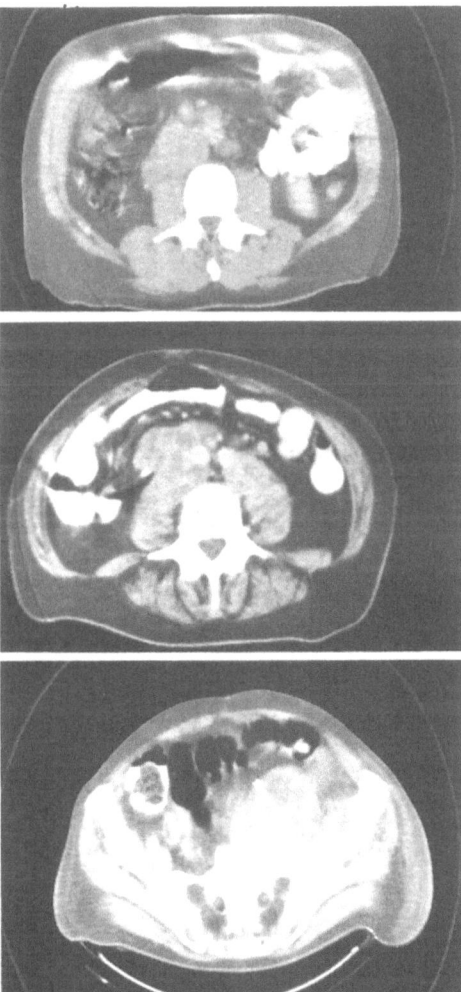

Fig. 6.10. Subdiaphragmatic NHL nodes (4 cm between the *two crosses*)

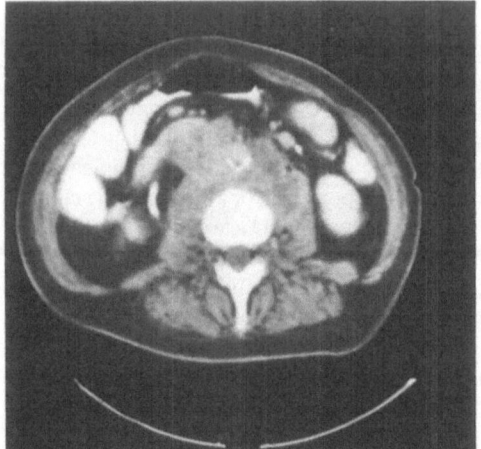

Solitary nodes between these limits are judged normal, whereas multiple nodes with diameters between 1 and 1.5 cm are considered pathologic [457]. It must also be remembered that lymphomatous nodes have a solid density, and are thus not enhanced by contrast material [70, 552]. The limitation of CT is related to lesion size: 5%–10% of HD patients have normal-sized pathologic nodes [347]. Likewise, diffuse nodal enlargement may be due to a reactive process rather than to lymphoma.

The sensitivity of CT scanning of the retroperitoneum is 65% for HD [121] and over 80% for

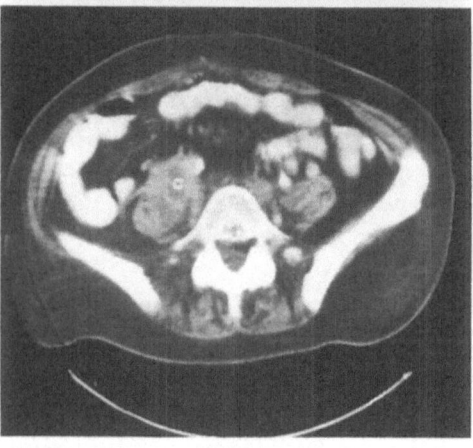

Fig. 6.11. Subdiaphragmatic NHL nodes with partial necrosis *(square)* at the level of the right primary iliac vein

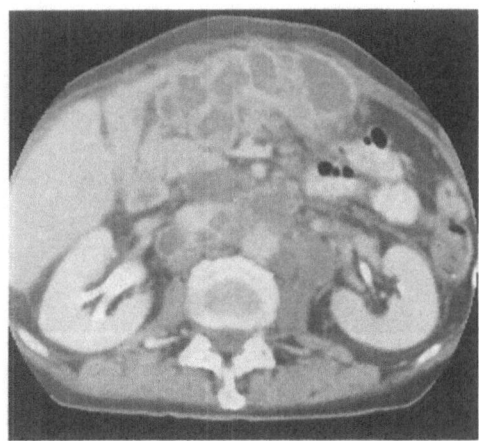

Fig. 6.13. Intra-and retroperitoneal NHL

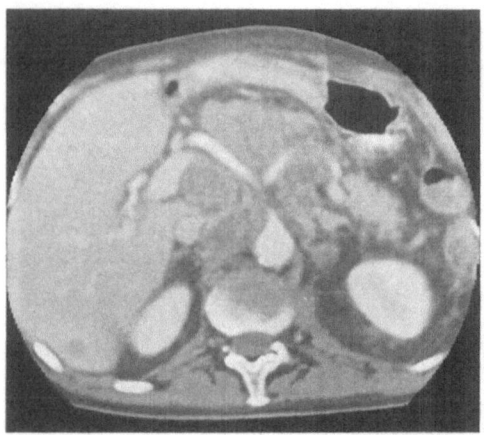

Fig. 6.12. Intra- and retroperitoneal NHL with involvement of the right hepatic lobe

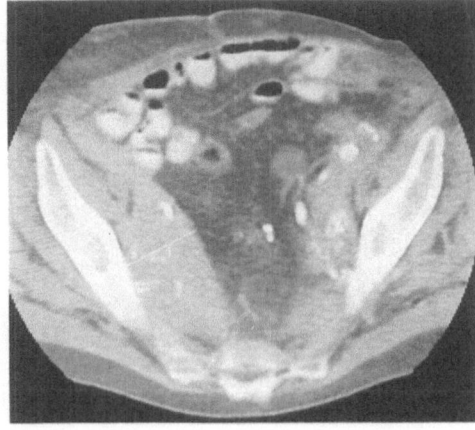

Fig. 6.14. Bilateral pelvic node NHL (CT performed 4 months after lymphography). *Line 1,* 43 mm

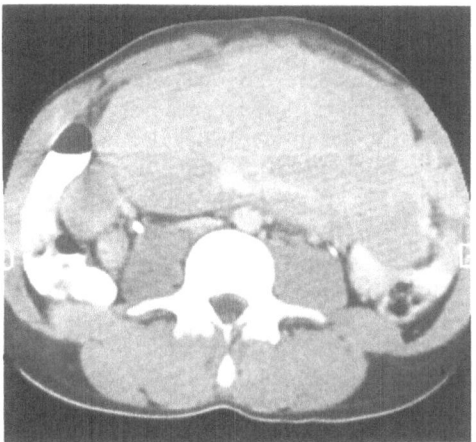

Fig. 6.15. Intraperitoneal NHL

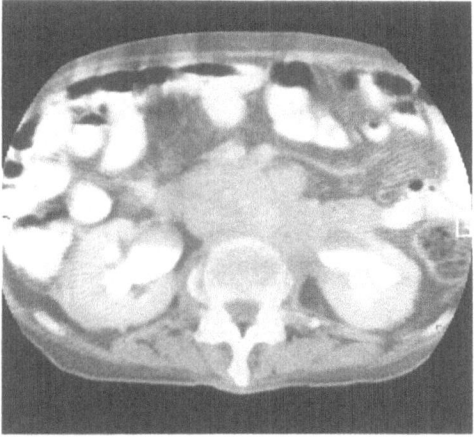

Fig. 6.16. Retroperitoneal NHL (90 HU in *square 1*) with bilateral renal stasis

NHL [149]; its specificity is 92% for HD and 86% for NHL [121, 149]. These figures give CT an overall accuracy of 75%-85% [121, 149, 319].

The utility of CT for monitoring response to therapy is underscored by the sensitivity of the technique in detecting recurrent disease, especially since half of all relapses are subclinical before they attain larger proportions [50, 458]. Serial CT scans are an easy means of comparing the status of nodal masses. Moreover, when doubt persists as to the fibrous or lymphomatous nature of a residual mass even after analysis of pre- and postcontrast density studies, CT can be used to guide one or more puncture biopsies in a search for lymphomatous elements [373, 378] (Figs. 6.17-6.19).

6.1.4 Radionuclide Studies

Gallium-67 citrate imaging has been extensively used for the study of lymphomas, and radionuclide studies correlate well with lymphography prior to treatment [91]. Despite the high incidence of equivocal results which is due to background radioactivity caused by intestinal excretion of the gallium isotope [91, 315], the sensitivity of gallium-67 studies can be improved by subtraction techniques [351]. Although 76% of treated NHL patients exhibit uptake in one or more lesions, the test is valid only when positive. The overall accuracy of ra-

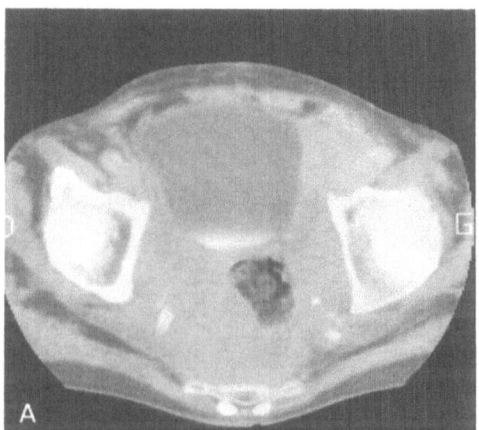

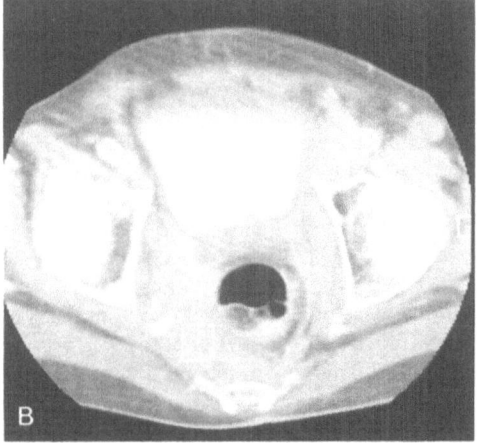

Fig. 6.17 A, B. Pelvic NHL (**A**) before and (**B**) after chemotherapy; persistence of lymphomatous tissue *(square 1)*

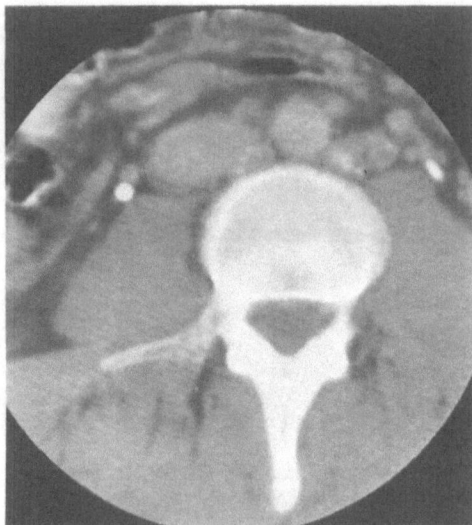

Fig. 6.18. Persistence of larger-than-normal nodes in a patient with treated HD. Guided biopsy was normal. Surveillance for over 2 years showing no changes allowed diagnosis of treatment-induced fibrosis

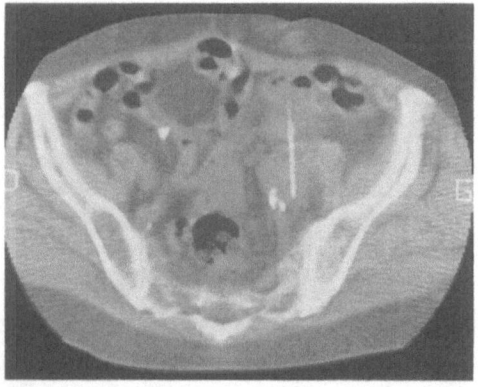

Fig. 6.19. Puncture biopsy of lymphomatous nodes misdiagnosed as treatment sequelae for 1 year: site prior to aspiration. Histological analysis revealed lymphomatous cells

dionuclide studies increases with nodal volume, from 46% for 1-cm nodes to 69% for 5-cm nodes [17]. This variation in accuracy as a function of lesion size explains the greater utility of such studies for NHL than for HD [543]. The sensitivity of gallium-67 citrate imaging is such that certain authors have suggested its use for the detection of relapses [315].

6.1.5 Interventional Imaging: Puncture Biopsy

Adenopathies are biopsied with 20- to 22-gauge needles; 18-gauge needles are preferable for tumor masses. Coagulation tests suffice before puncture, and the procedure can be performed even on an outpatient basis. Lymphography, ultrasonography, and CT can all be used for guidance purposes [241, 400, 681]. While the technique gives no false-positives [400, 681], its overall accuracy is only 64%, since there are few cases in which a definite diagnosis is possible. Moreover, the small amount of tissue obtained by percutaneous biopsy precludes diagnosis of nodular disease.

Nevertheless, puncture biopsy remains extremely useful for the detection of recurrent disease and especially for the analysis of residual masses after therapy. Even though biopsies are valid only when positive, the absence of lymphomatous tissue in a residual mass biopsy should lead to modification of the therapeutic strategy. Laparotomy remains indispensable in certain cases, but guided puncture biopsy can often correct a presumptive diagnosis, and it has the added advantage of causing few complications.

6.2 Exploratory Strategy for Abdominal Lymph Nodes

The optimum investigative approach differs for HD and NHL, as technological advances in CT have modified the diagnostic potential of this technique for abdominal NHL nodes [119, 120]. Until such time as the contributions of magnetic resonance imaging (MRI; Fig. 6.20) are defined, certain points must be borne in mind: lymphography is irreplaceable for detailed node analysis, but can only examine the retroperitoneum. It cannot analyze the celiomesenteric nodes which are involved in nearly 50% of cases of NHL, although rarely (4%) in HD.

The cost of the various imaging modalities varies considerably. Plain abdominal films used for surveillance after lymphography are inexpensive when compared to CT. The cost of diagnostic ultrasound varies from country to country; in France, a sonogram costs 70% less than a CT scan.

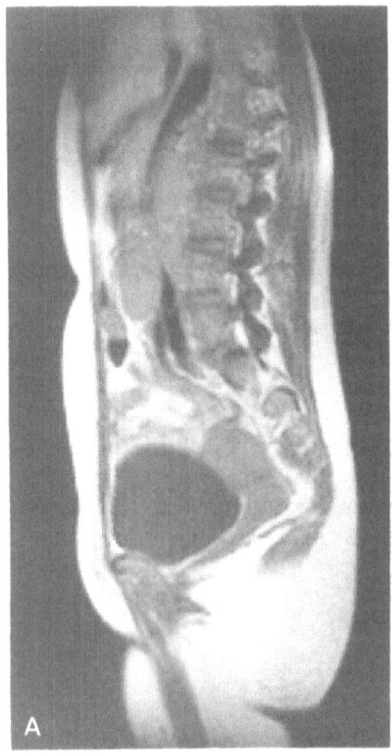

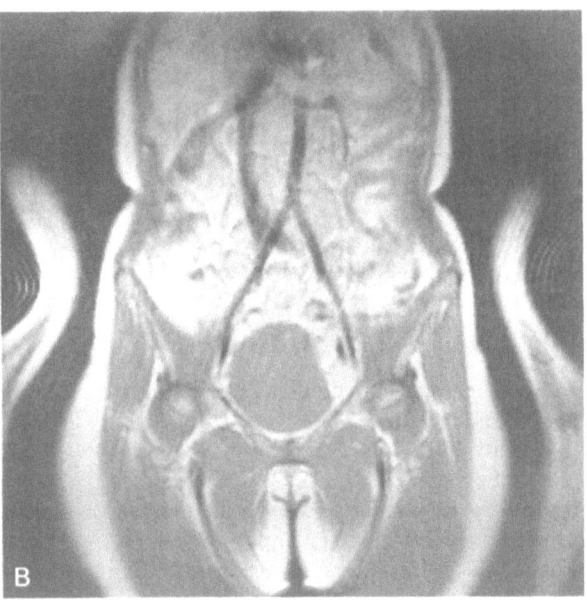

◁ **Fig. 6.20 A, B.** Retroperitoneal NHL nodes visualized by magnetic resonance imaging (MRI). **A** Lateral view; **B** frontal view

6.2.1 Hodgkin's Disease

Nodes affected by HD may be normal in size and present only structural abnormalities. In addition, celiomesenteric involvement is rare. These facts make lymphography the preferred investigative procedure. Castellino [121] has even reported lympography to have a 70% greater diagnostic value than CT. When dealing with a suspicious normal-sized node, lymphography-guided biopsy should allow diagnosis.

Patient follow-up warrants particular attention. The amount of residual contrast material after 18 months is insufficient for correct surveillance in two-thirds of cases [192, 593]. Furthermore, 95% of HD relapses occur within 3 years, and 30% of these recurrences involve the retroperitoneum. Half of these retroperitioneal relapses are subclinical [112]. In view of these characteristics of HD relapses, a second lymphography is warranted as soon as the contrast material has been resorbed. This measure ensures maximum efficacy of retroperitoneal surveillance during HD. Lymphography can al-ways be completed by ultrasonographic exploration of the celiomesenteric region, the spleen, and the liver. The indications for CT in HD generally appear limited to those cases in which lymphography is insufficient or equivocal.

6.2.2 Non-Hodgkin's Lymphomas

Since NHL nodes are often bulky and nearly half of all patients have celiomesenteric involvement, CT is the imaging modality of choice. When only one or a few nodes with a diameter between 1 and 1.5 cm are found, lymphography can be performed to obtain morphological data on nodal structure. CT has the additional advantage of being the technique which best defines the extent of disease, thus allowing appropriate therapeutic decisions.

CT is justified for the surveillance of patients with NHL if 6-month intervals are acceptable. When shorter intervals are required, particularly for the lower peritoneal and iliac regions, which are poorly analyzed by ultrasound, lymphography is advisable, since plain abdominal films can be used for follow-up purposes [183, 368].

7 Gastrointestinal Lymphomas

J.-N. Bruneton, J.-J. Manzino, and E. Caramella

The digestive tract, liver, spleen, biliary tract, and pancreas can all be affected by lymphomas. Barium studies remain useful for investigation of the digestive tract. The radiological features suggestive of lymphoma prior to histological confirmation, which remains indispensable, have been compiled from the extensive data in the many relevant studies published on the subject. By contrast, not even the most recent radiological techniques appear to have improved the efficacy of imaging in detecting lymphomas of the spleen or liver.

7.1 Malignant Lymphomas of the Gastrointestinal Tract

Malignant lymphomas of the gastrointestinal tract have been the subject of numerous recent studies aimed at defining the radiological appearances of these rare entities, and in particular the non-Hodgkin's lymphomas (NHL). Owing to the submucosal origin of the disease, even deep biopsies performed with state-of-the-art techniques are not always positive. This explains the continued importance of barium studies, especially since therapeutic approaches have evolved. As an example, surgery is no longer the treatment of choice for disease sites in the stomach, the most frequent site of gastrointestinal lymphoma, as many authors now advocate radiotherapy and above all chemotherapy. Furthermore, computed tomography (CT) and ultrasonography now allow improved evaluation of subdiaphragmatic nodes and the extent of disease within the gastrointestinal tract [367].

The radiological features of gastrointestinal tract NHL and Hodgkin's disease (HD) warrant differentiation because of the differences in their patterns of anatomical distribution and frequency. Nearly one in every 20 cases of NHL is a primary gastrointestinal site with a favorable prognosis.

In contrast to carcinomas, NHL generally does not induce any fibroblastic stroma reaction. The resultant large lesions are readily demonstrated radiologically, and despite the frequent absence of clinical signs, their size suggests the correct diagnosis. Both primary and secondary HD are rare, and in contrast to NHL their prognosis is poor, as they correspond to stage IV disease from the outset. HD is associated with an intense fibroblastic stroma reaction causing moderate-sized focal lesions suggestive of carcinoma.

7.1.1 Non-Hodgkin's Lymphoma

The overall frequency of primary NHL of the gastrointestinal tract has been evaluated at 5% to 6.2% [75, 212, 534, 556]. The incidence reported for secondary forms is even higher, ranging from 15.6% [556] to 44% [534], depending on whether radiological/clinical data [556] or autopsy series [534] are presented. For Dawson [154], diagnosis of primary gastrointestinal lymphomas rests on four criteria:

No enlargement of peripheral or mediastinal lymph nodes
Normal white blood cell counts
Predominance of the gastrointestinal lesion, with only regional lymph node involvement
No liver or spleen involvement

Primary lymphomas are often considered focal lesions, corresponding to one of four stages [445]:

Stage I: submucosal involvement with invasion toward the mucosa
Stage II: parietal involvement, but no node enlargement

Stage III: lesions involving the entire wall plus associated node enlargement

Stage IV: generalized disease

The radiological appearances of primary and secondary lymphomas are similar, with the exception of those affecting the colon [363]. The prognosis for primary forms varies from 30% to 45% survival at 5 years [63], and is thus better than for carcinoma.

7.1.1.1. Esophagus

The rarity of esophageal involvement is underscored by the fact that only 15 cases were found in a literature review of 2200 cases of gastrointestinal NHL [45, 101, 107, 465]. NHL of the esophagus represents less than 1% of all gastrointestinal lymphomas (Table 7.1). Dissemination from mediastinal nodes and extension of a gastric lymphoma into the lower third of the esophagus are most frequent [292]. Clinical symptoms were cited in only half of the cases reviewed, with dysphagia being mentioned in only 50% of those.

Lesions are generally demonstrated radiologically as nodular masses; multiple nodules (Fig. 7.1) are more prevalent than solitary ones, and they are almost always associated with a gastric lesion of the same type. The differential diagnoses for nodular lesions include leiomyoma (although NHL is usually more extensive), esophageal varices (but varices tend to have a tortuous appearance), and hematogenous metastases (espicially of malignant melanoma). Less frequent findings include large ulcerations [101, 107] and infiltrative processes, which on rare occasions can cause obstructive stenosis. In these last cases, radiological images can return to normal following radiotherapy.

7.1.1.2 Stomach

The stomach is the most frequent site of gastrointestinal NHL; this is particularly true of primary forms. For Freeman [212], gastric sites are the origin of NHL in 3.9% of cases. Other authors have reported a frequency as high as 6% [88, 511]. Gastric disease sites predominate among gastrointestinal tract lesions in general, accounting for 48.2%–78.5% of cases [88, 181, 389, 645]. NHL of the stomach represents 40%–75% of gastric sarcomas [85, 139] and 3%–5% of all gastric neoplasms [344, 570] (Table 7.1).

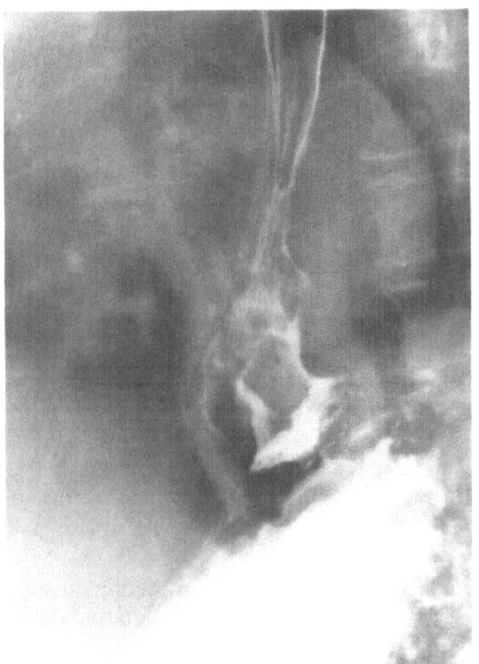

Fig. 7.1 NHL of the esophagus: multinodular pattern (associated with gastric NHL)

Table 7.1. Incidence of NHL of the digestive tract

	Esophagus (%)	Stomach (%)	Small bowel (%)	Colon/rectum (%)
Incidence of primary forms [212]	0.03	3.9	1.2	0.9
Incidence with respect to other digestive tract segments	<1	50–70	35–70	15
Incidence with respect to other malignant tumors	Rare	3–5	10–30	0.5

Some 1100 clinical reports were reviewed in the literature [36, 54, 85, 88, 139, 141, 205, 209, 211, 214, 217, 248, 253, 254, 277, 285, 292, 296, 321, 364, 365, 367, 369, 377, 389, 402, 422, 428, 448, 470, 511, 548, 566, 569, 570, 586, 587, 611, 616]. The average patient age was 59 years; 65% of patients were male. Table 7.2 summarizes the frequencies of clinical symptoms. Dysphagia was rare (2.1% of cases) and associated with involvement of the upper third of the stomach, with or without extension to the esophagus. Signs of perforation were present in 3.6% of cases. The site of predilection is the antrum (62.7%) [364]. Owing to the absence of a fibroblastic stroma reaction, lesions attained 10 cm or more in two-thirds of cases [321, 402, 428, 570].

Radiological examinations, and barium studies in particular, are essential, since the submucosal nature of these lesions often precludes detection by endoscopy, even though this last technique diagnoses malignancy in 88% of cases [248, 369, 587]. Biopsy provides the diagnosis in 27%-67% of NHL cases [248, 471, 587, 616, 675]. On rare occasions, adenocarcinomas have been observed to develop from lymphomatous gastric lesions [569].

The prognosis for gastric NHL is twice as favorable as that for cancer; the overall survival rate at 5 years is now 24%, vs only 10.5% before 1952 [139, 214, 288, 422]. The survival rate ranges from 42% to 68% for focal disease [63, 185, 321, 448], but is only 17.4% for diffuse lesions.

Radiological Features. Barium studies are especially important, owing to the limitations of endoscopy. Table 7.3 lists the radiological features compiled from a review of 570 cases (Figs. 7.2-7.7). The raritiy of stenotic forms in the stomach is related to the absence of a fibroblastic stroma reaction. Combined forms exist in 28% of cases, and 14.7% of them include diffuse gastric disease [141, 248, 292]. While a lesion in the antrum, the site of predilection, is nondiagnostic by itself, lesion size (10 cm or more) is suggestive of NHL before histological confirmation, even though there may be few clinical signs. Both Meyers [431] and Hricak [292] have cited extragastric extension as another characteristic of the disease. According to Hricak, extension to the esophagus occurs in 10% of cases, and spread to the duodenum is even more frequent (33%) [292].

The radiological appearance of gastric NHL is useful for differential diagnosis, since cancer is

Table 7.2. Incidence of clinical symptoms in gastric, intestinal, and colorectal NHL

Clinical symptom	Stomach (1100 cases) (%)	Intestine (700 cases) (%)	Colon/rectum (400 cases) (%)
Pain	73	63	74
Weight loss	41	34	57
Bleeding	26	24	28
Vomiting	24	15	11
Diarrhea	-	20	43.6
Palpable mass	18	54	40
Obstruction	-	15	22

Table 7.3. Incidence of radiological patterns in gastric, intestinal, and colorectal NHL: radiological diagnosis

Radiological pattern	Stomach (570 cases) (%)	Small bowel (200 cases) (%)	Colon (118 cases) (%)
Ulcerated form	49	33.5	3.5
Tumoral form (>3 cm diameter)	36	43	50
Infiltrating form:		53	
– non-stenosing	22	33 (aneurysmal form in 17%)	25.5
– stenosing		20	
Hypertrophic form	19		
Nodular form (<3 cm diameter)	2	4.5	45.5
Frequency of combined forms	28	34	24.5
Radiological diagnosis of:			
– NHL	13	30	0
– malignancy	77	20-50	50-70

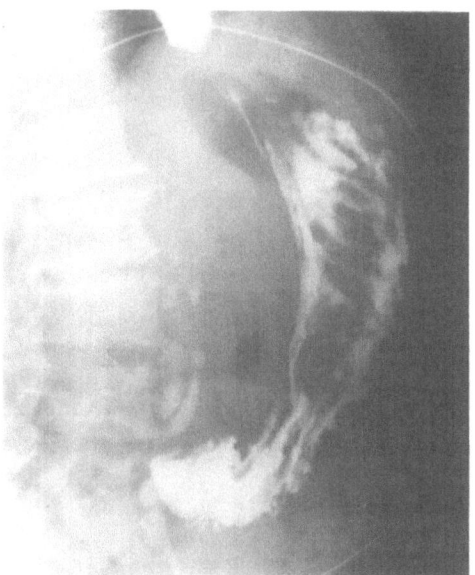

Fig. 7.2. NHL of the stomach: diffuse hypertrophy of the folds

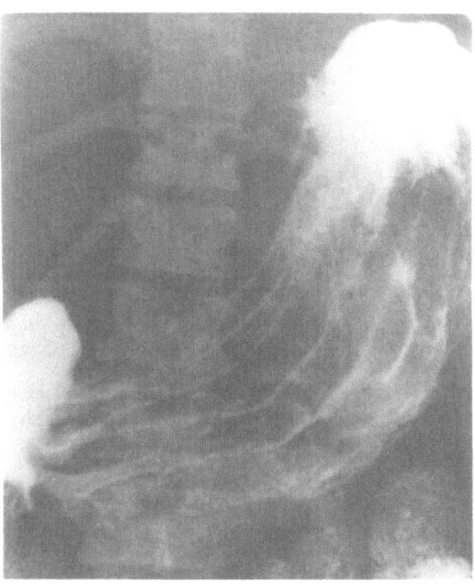

Fig. 7.3 NHL of the stomach: diffuse hypertrophy of the folds

often hard to exclude solely on the basis of symptomatology. Hypertrophic folds are suggestive of benign segmental or diffuse hypertrophy, or Ménétrier's disease [418]. Less frequently, gastric ulcer is entertained as a possibility for benign-appearing filling defects. Nodular lesions, often contiguous to a tumoral mass, can suggest other gastric sarcomas [96, 549]. Benign lymphoid hyperplasia can resemble gastric NHL clinically and radiologically [122, 253, 301, 425, 492]. The criteria for diagnosis of lymphoid hyperplasia are purely histological: existence of true germinal formations, presence of a polymorphous inflammatory infiltrate, and absence of lymphomatous node involvement.

Barium studies have a diagnostic accuracy of 77% for malignancy and 13% for lymphoma. In very large series, the lymphoma detection rate has even reached 56% [675]. Arteriography appears of limited value for the investigation of gastric lymphomas, except for the detection of moderate hypervascularity and arteriolar abnormalities [217]. By contrast, ultrasonography offers two advantages [548]: (a) detection of gastric wall thickening, which corresponds to submucosal infiltration and is visualized as a solid but highly hypoechoic or even fluid-ap-

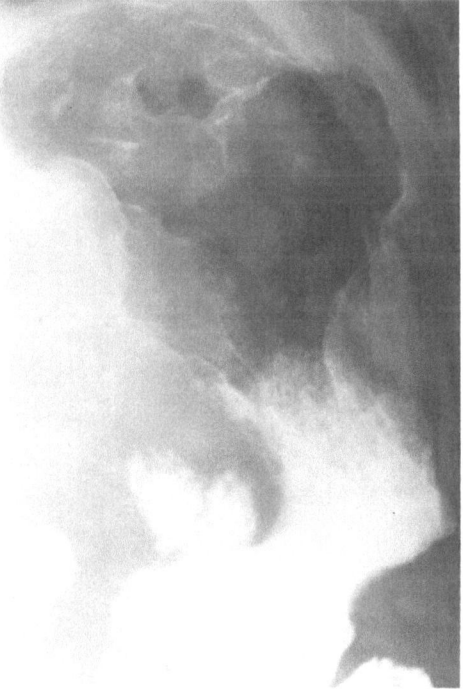

Fig. 7.4. NHL of the stomach: combined form (hypertrophy of the folds and ulceration)

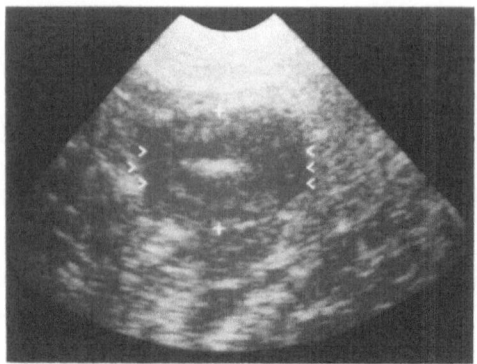

Fig. 7.5. NHL of the stomach: gastric wall thickening *(arrowheads)* demonstrated by ultrasonography. (Oblique section: 24 mm between the *two crosses*)

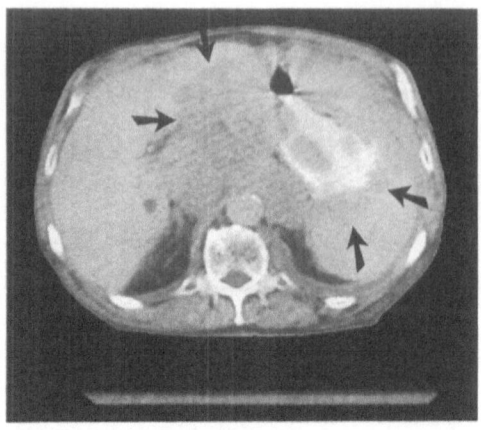

Fig. 7.7. NHL of the stomach: diffuse thickening *(arrows)* of the gastric wall

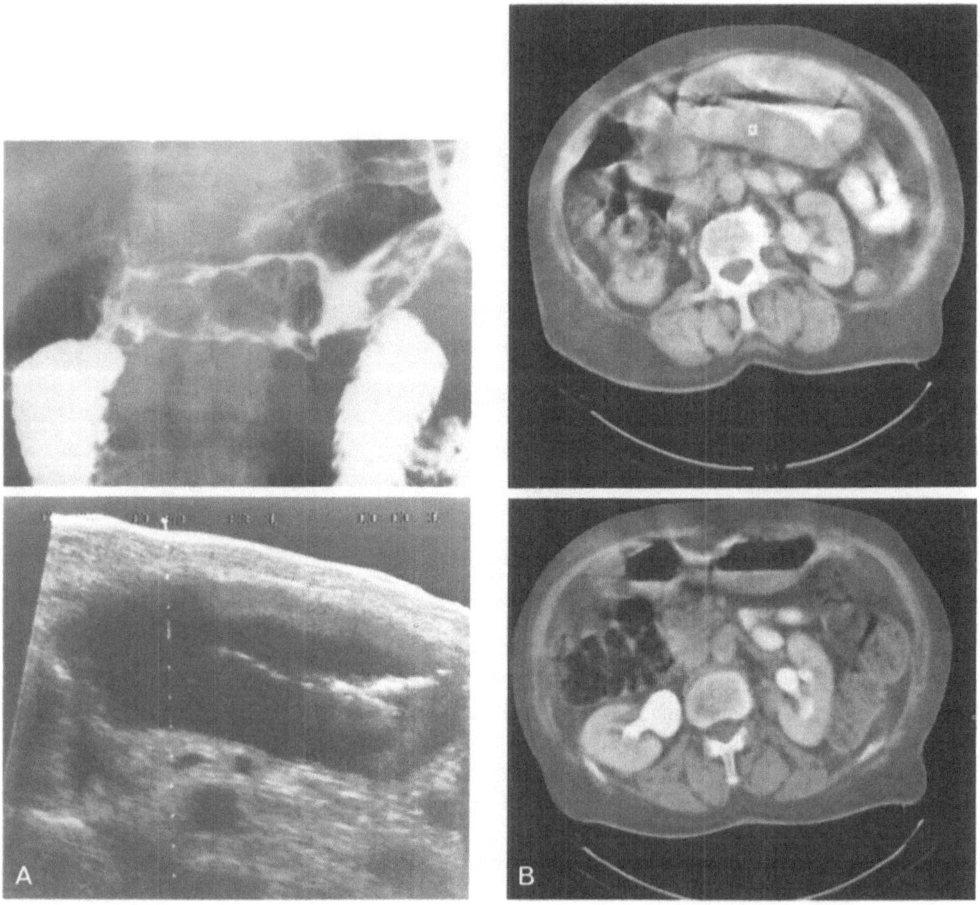

Fig. 7.6 A, B. NHL of the stomach: barium study. **A** Ultrasound and **B** CT findings: wall thickening *(square)* and ulceration

pearing pattern, and (b) detection of celiomesenteric and retroperitoneal adenopathies as part of disease extension work-ups. The examination of choice for pretherapy work-ups of gastric lymphoma is CT [89]; moreover, CT can be performed even when meteorism makes ultrasound impractical. In addition to visualizing retroperitoneal nodes, CT can demonstrate localized wall thickening or disease extension to regional nodes or neighboring viscera [367]. Gallium-67 studies appear restricted to patient surveillance during treatment [296].

Gastric NHL can thus be diagnosed by barium contrast radiography completed by CT or ultrasonography, keeping in mind the following general features:

Radiological lesions at least 10 cm in diameter in over two-thirds of cases.
Lack of correlation between often discrete clinical symptoms and large radiological lesions
The rarity of stenotic forms
The frequency of complex forms, which can involve extension to the esophagus and especially to the duodenum

7.1.1.3 Small Bowel

The second most frequent site of gastrointestinal NHL is the small intestine [141, 212, 248, 316, 471, 616] (Table 7.1). Since multiple gastrointestinal disease sites are common, involvement of the small intestine occurs in 35%–50% of all patients with gastrointestinal lymphomas [367]. Primary NHL accounts for 10%–40% of all small-bowel neoplasms [12, 50]. There is apparently a significant geographical factor, particularly in the Far East, where small-bowel lesions are the most common primary gastrointestinal NHL, as well as being the most frequent malignancy of the small intestine [124]. The general characteristics of these lesions were drawn from a review of some 700 cases in the literature [11, 63, 65, 138, 141, 150, 176, 211, 248, 277, 286, 363, 377, 420, 435, 471, 479, 482, 493, 514, 564, 616, 633, 636]. The average patient age was 47 years; 57% of patients were male. Table 7.2 lists the associated clinical symptoms. The palpable mass noted in 54% of patients corresponded either to the lymphomatous lesion itself or to stasis above a tumoral

site causing obstruction. Obstruction occurred in 15% of cases, perforation in 14.5% [141, 616, 633], and malabsorption in 7% [150, 215, 248, 298, 299, 377, 389, 590, 602]. Development of lymphoma as a complication of celiac disease is also a rare possibility [138, 493].
Burkitt's lymphoma, which generally affects persons under the age of 30, is invariably accompanied by symptoms which include diarrhea and absorption disorders. The entire small intestine is involved, although the terminal ileum is often spared. The gastrointestinal tract is affected much more frequently by Burkitt's lymphoma than by other forms of NHL [176, 449, 514, 547]. The majority of lesions occur in the ileum (68%) [411, 446], but both the jejunum (38%) and duodenum (12%) can also be affected [23, 99, 150, 389]. Multiple disease sites occur in different segments (18%) or in the same segment (16%) of the small intestine in 34% of patients [363]. Lesions exceed 5 cm in over 77% of cases; smaller lesions correspond to focal constricting or multinodular disease.
Although the overall prognosis for primary NHL of the intestine is comparable to that for gastric lymphomas [88, 446], association with an immunoproliferative small-intestine disease carries a poor prognosis [636].

Radiological Features. Table 7.3 lists the frequencies of radiological forms based on 200 cases in the literature [73, 85, 117, 150, 215, 299, 389, 468, 602]. Infiltrative forms predominate (Figs. 7.8–7.13), representing over one half of all cases (53%). Owing to the absence of a fibroblastic stroma reaction, the lumen is generally dilated because of the destructive action of the tumor; constricting lesions are less common. The most frequent radiological findings are nonconstricting lesions with thickened folds, occasionally with a pseudonodular appearance or loss of the mucous membrane pattern, or with a classical aneurysmal appearance (17%). Aneurysmal forms are suggestive of NHL; radiologically, these lesions have been compared to a length of garden hose whose supra- and subjacent segments seem normal [468]. Aneurysmal lesions can attain considerable sizes. The distal loop cannot be opacified until relatively late in the examination, owing to the large dimensions of the lesion and the loss of peristaltic capacity. Lumen dilatation is

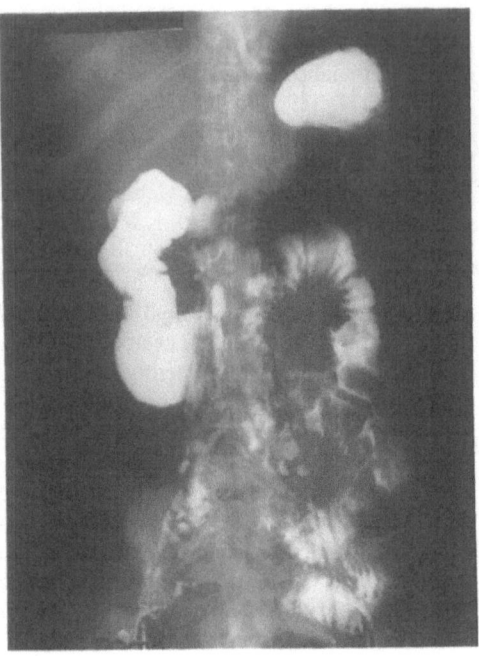

Fig. 7.8. NHL of the jejunum: infiltrative form

variable. On early films, the barium has a mottled appearance, corresponding to secretions and food particles trapped in the dilated loop. Both segmental dilatation near a fibrous or neoplastic inflammatory zone and scleroderma (which causes dilatation but is characterized by long atonic segments with atrophic connivent valvulae) can be ruled out because of the complete disappearance of the connivent valvulae. In rare instances, however, conjunctive sarcomas have a similar radiological appearance. Infiltrative growths are an infrequent cause of lumen narrowing; 9.1% of these growths are constricting multinodular tumors, while 10.9% are ulcerative forms associated with loss of mucosal markings. The differential diagnosis for focal lesions is carcinoma. When large segments of intestine appear involved, confusion is possible with peritoneal carcinosis.

Tumoral lesions, accounting for 43% of intestinal NHL, present in a variety of forms: extraluminal mass (22.5%), intramural tumor or intraluminal mass (18%), and "dumbbell" tumor (2.5%).

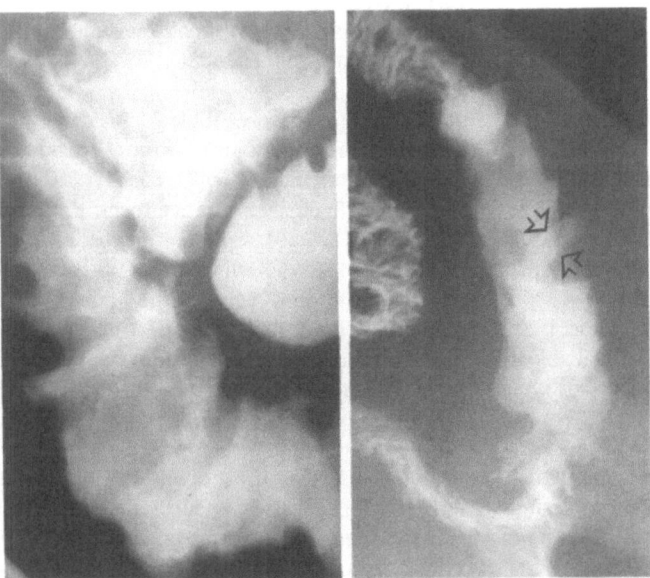

Fig. 7.9. NHL of the small intestine: infiltrative form, complicated in the *righthand* case by ulceration *(arrows)*

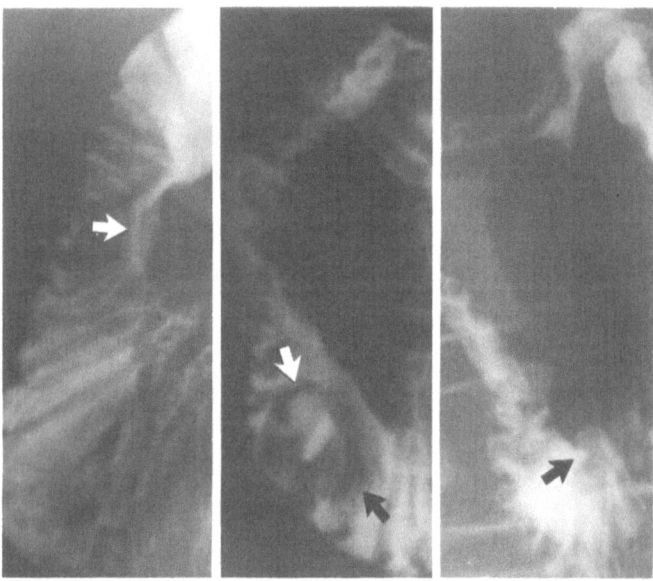

Fig. 7.10. NHL of the duodenum: ulcerated forms *(arrows)* in three different patients

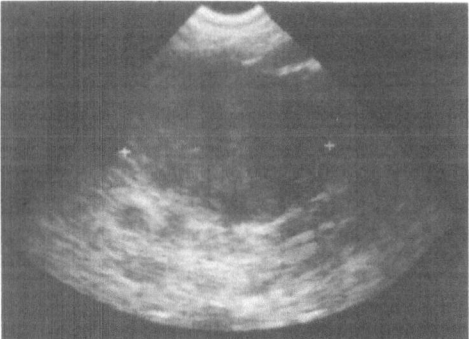

Fig. 7.11. Duodenojejunal NHL: pseudoaneurysmal form visualized by ultrasound. (Transverse scan: 75 mm between the *two crosses*)

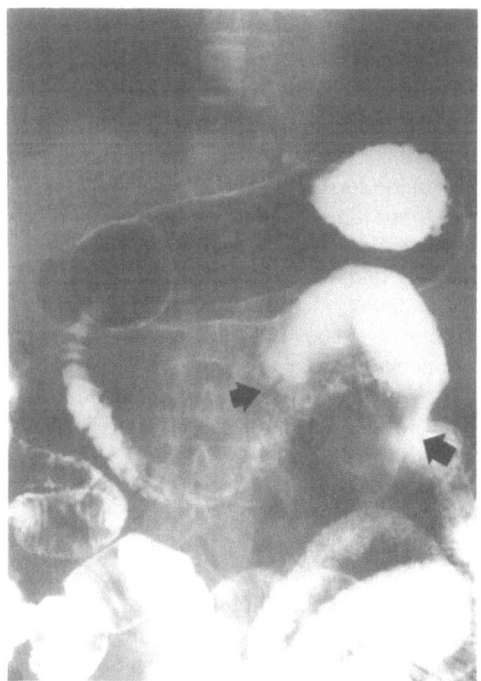

Fig. 7.12. Duodenojejunal NHL: pseudoaneurysmal ▷ form *(arrows)* demonstrated by a barium examination

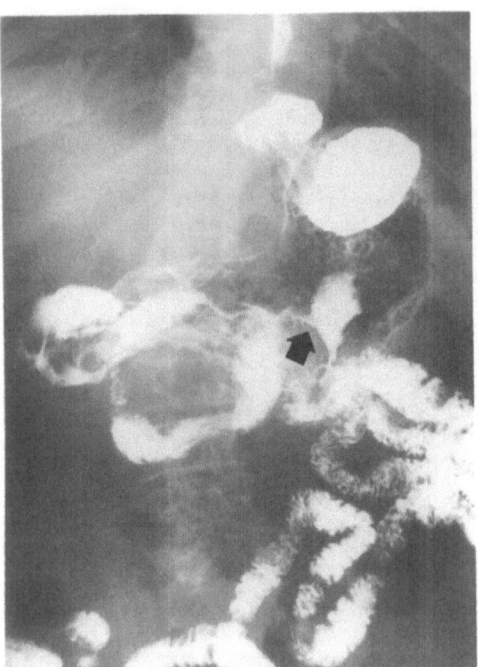

Fig. 7.13. Duodenojejunal NHL: pseudoaneurysmal and ulcerated form *(arrow)*

In cases of predominant mesenteric extraluminal masses, a further distinction is made between nodal forms and sprue. In nodal forms, an extrinsic mass syndrome is provoked by mesenteric adenopathies that displace the adjacent loops. Sprue patterns, observed in 10.1% of cases [419], are always clinically signalled by diarrhea, and in 30% of patients by steatorrhea. The radiological features associated with extraluminal masses include dilated loops with prominent mucosa and signs of flocculation and segmentation. Both intramural and intraluminal forms cause obstruction, and especially intussusception, owing to their large size (5-7 cm long). Intra-extraluminal (dumbbell) forms are much rarer, but can cause fistulization in adjacent loops. Ulcerating lesions (33.5% of cases) are frequently associated with infiltrating and multinodular forms.

Nodular lesions are generally multiple; less than 3 cm in diameter, they show up as numerous filling defects, and the mucosa projects upward and appears "studded." The lumen is not narrowed by these rare forms, which account for only 4.5% of cases. The differential diagno-

sis is regional enteritis. Nodular lesions are often encountered in Burkitt's lymphoma [514].

Of the review cases, 34% mentioned the simultaneous presence of various combinations of these radiological forms. Diffuse multinodular forms, which can involve the entire gastrointestinal tract, are extremely rare [155, 266, 496]. Radiologically complex forms generally cause obstruction (9.5% of cases, including 6% for intussusception). The frequencies reported by radiological studies were lower than those for clinical investigations, since barium studies (not even a barium enema) are not always performed when there are clinical symptoms of obstruction. Fistulas, observed in 1.7% of cases, are generally associated with dumbbell tumors. Perforation was noted in 5% of cases. Radiological exploration of complex forms was often limited to an abdominal plain film.

Radiological studies are responsible for diagnosing malignancy in 20%-50% of cases and lymphoma in 30% [389]. Less frequent diagnoses before histological confirmation include regional enteritis [196] and polyposis. As for investigations of the stomach, various other techniques have been proposed. Angiography is rarely used [39, 55, 270, 396], and shows avascular lesions without neovascularity or venous phase abnormalities. This technique appears of no utility for the diagnosis of small-bowel NHL. CT [479] detects tumoral masses and can define their relations to adjacent loops and, above all, to the retroperitoneum. This is helpful when the purely intestinal origin of a tumor cannot be formally established on the basis of contrast radiography. Ultrasonography can visualize a thickened bowel wall, which will often be strongly hypoechoic or even cystlike [435]. In the rare instances when hypoechoic patterns are absent, only a thickened wall is seen [442].

7.1.1.4 Colon and Rectum

Primary NHL of the colon and rectum is rare, representing only 0.1% of all cases of NHL [212]. Colorectal sites follow gastric and intestinal sites in frequency, and account for an average of 15% of cases (Table 7.1). Lymphoma is exceptional, though, being the cause of only 0.5% of all malignant tumors of the colon and rectum [679].

Nearly 400 cases were reviewed to define the general features of colorectal NHL [44, 79, 133, 141, 142, 145, 154, 159, 162, 180, 209, 211, 242, 248, 261, 277, 283, 302, 325, 363, 377, 389, 446, 452, 471, 472, 474, 488, 496, 503, 526, 540, 545, 564, 573, 602, 628, 639, 650, 667]. The average patient age was 50 years, with a range of 3–82 years; 64% of patients were male. Patients with primary lesions were generally younger than those with secondary colorectal involvement [277]. The average age of patients with primary ileocecal lesions was much lower, around 30 years [277, 377].

Table 7.2 summarizes the associated clinical symptoms. Palpable masses, a frequent finding noted in 40% of patients, corresponded either to the tumor or to stercoral stasis above a stenotic area. As for gastric and intestinal NHL, asymptomatic involvement was rare, especially with secondary forms. This is in contradiction to autopsy finding [474]. NHL can develop as a complication of hemorrhagic rectocolitis [545, 653], while lymphomatous colonic lesions may be complicated by colonic pneumatosis or acute colectasia [472].

The sites of colonic NHL, in decreasing order of frequency, are the cecum (52.5% of cases), rectum (21.2%), right colon (13.8%), left colon (13.5%), and transverse colon (5.6%). Concomitant ileal involvement exists in 38% of cases of primary NHL of the colon [44, 145, 180, 277, 667].

Except for pseudopolypoid forms, primary lesions have an average diameter of over 5 cm (8 cm for Wychulis [667]). Diffuse, often nodular, forms usually range from 2 mm to 2.5 cm. The prognosis for primary forms (34%–55.2% survival at 5 years) contrasts markedly with the unfavorable outlook for secondary involvement (less than 1 year for all authors) [277, 667].

Radiological Features. Table 7.3 summarizes the appearances reported in 118 review cases, either alone or in combination (Fig. 7.14–7.17). Tumors (intramural or intraluminal, dumbbell, and purely mesenteric forms) were the most frequent type of lesion (50%). Intraluminal tumors, the most prevalent (30%), are a common cause of obstruction (with or without intussusception), owing to their average size of 5–10 cm. These tumors are generally primary lesions [242, 446, 472, 602], and the usual diagnosis based on radiological findings is carcinoma. Dumbbell forms, which account for 19% of cases, are also frequently misdiagnosed as carcinoma. Purely mesenteric forms represent only 1% of cases.

Small intramural or intraluminal nodular lesions are responsible for 45.5% of cases; these often multiple forms can attain 2.5 cm in diameter and be misdiagnosed as ulcerative colitis, Crohn's disease, amibiasis, or pseudomembranous colitis. Smaller lesions may be mistaken for polyposis or lymphoid hypertrophy [162, 377, 564, 674].

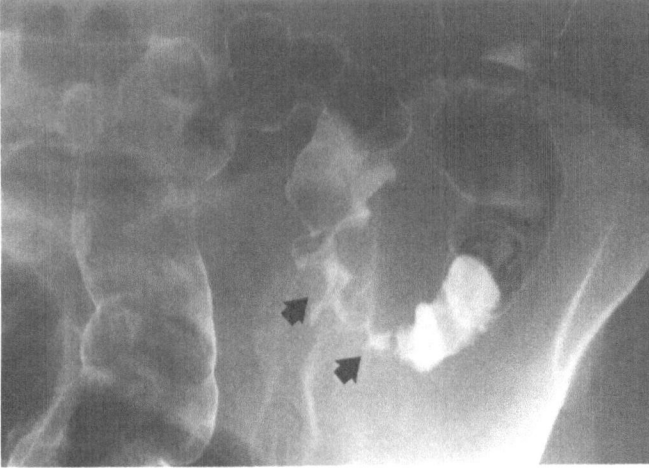

Fig. 7.14. NHL of the colon: infiltrating form *(arrows)*

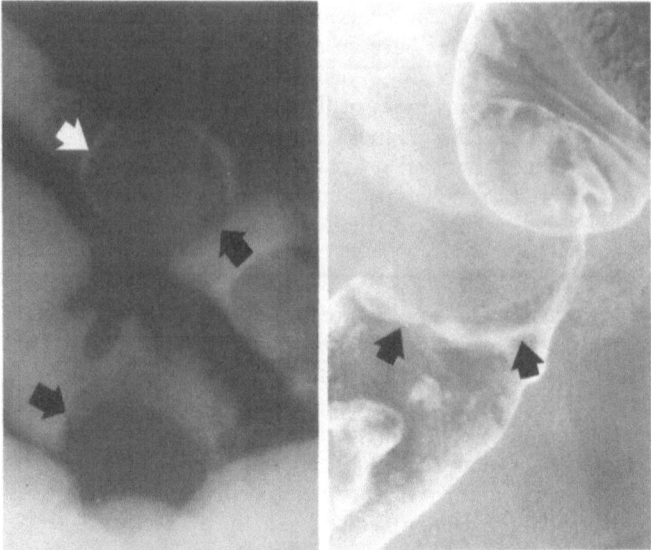

Fig. 7.15. NHL of the colon: tumoral forms *(arrows)* in two different patients

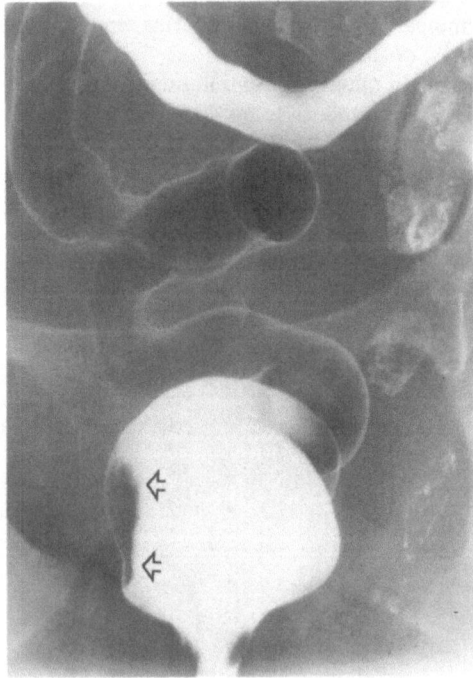

Fig. 7.16. NHL of the rectum: intramural form *(arrows)*

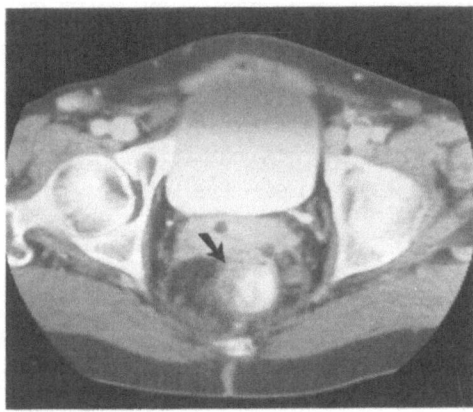

Fig. 7.17. NHL of the rectum: intramural form *(arrow)*

Diffuse or focal infiltrating lesions represent 25.5% of cases. The differential diagnosis is an inflammatory lesion or, when the sigmoid is involved, a gynecological pathology [674].

Ulcerating forms are rare in the colon, accounting for only 3.5% of cases. Complex radiological patterns are observed in 24.5% of patients. In contrast to gastric and small-bowel lymphomas, the radiological appearances of colonic NHL differ for primary forms (essentially tumors) and secondary involvement (usually multinodular or infiltrating lesions). The most frequent primary form in the rectum is an infiltrating lesion with thickened folds [446, 488, 602]; nodular forms are less common.

Radiological studies thus appear insufficient for the diagnosis of primary colonic or rectal NHL. The occurrence of tumoral forms, however, explains the diagnosis of malignancy in 50%–70% of cases.

7.1.2 Hodgkin's Disease

Both primary and secondary HD are much less frequent than NHL of the gastrointestinal tract. HD represents only 1.5%–1.7% of all malignant lymphomas of the digestive tract [299, 377]. In the series of Novak [470], gastrointestinal sites represented only 1.2% of all cases of HD. For Portmann [507], all primary and secondary clinical forms in the gastrointestinal tract accounted for 3.7% of cases.

In addition to the limited involvement of the gastrointestinal tract, HD differs from NHL on a histological level, since it induces a fibroblastic stroma reaction. Although the resultant lesions are relatively focal, even primary gastrointestinal sites of HD have a poor prognosis, being considered stage IV disease from the outset. While the rarity of this pathology precludes any general statements as to prognosis, gastrointestinal HD appears to have a less favorable outcome than gastrointestinal NHL.

7.1.2.1 Esophagus

The esophagus is the least frequent site of gastrointestinal HD [71, 289, 662]. Few reports of primary lesions have been published in the literature [101, 148, 439, 491, 560, 575, 620]. The average patient age is relatively low (38 years in review cases). Clinical symptoms almost always include dysphagia; weight loss and pain are less common. Totally asymptomatic cases and achalasia are exceptional [491].

By contrast with other gastrointestinal sites of HD, esophageal lesions tend to be large, ranging from 5 to 10 cm in diameter. There do not appear to be any sites of predilection within the esophagus itself. Radiotherapy has always been reported to cause a regression in lesion size [148, 439, 560, 575, 620].

Radiological findings include neoplastic-appearing esophageal narrowing, considered cancerous before confirmation; intramural masses suggesting a benign process, for which the differential diagnosis is leiomyoma or metastasis; and multiple polypoid masses that may appear varicoid. Diagnosis of HD is possible only after histological examination.

7.1.2.2 Stomach

The general characteristics of gastric HD were defined after the review of 89 literature cases [52, 58, 71, 160, 203, 209, 219, 229, 275, 285, 412, 420, 470, 507]. As indicated in Table 7.4, the stomach is the most common site of gastrointestinal HD [71, 289, 662]. Autopsies following generalized lymphoma have demonstrated at least microscopic evidence of gastric involvement in one in every ten cases. HD accounts for 0.5% of all gastric neoplasms [421] and 5.6% of all gastric malignant lymphomas [145, 325, 463, 549, 570]. Common presenting complaints, in decreasing order of frequency, include abdominal pain (67.4% of cases), weight loss (50.6%), anorexia (25.8%), and nausea and vomiting (24.7%).

Lesions are less than or equal to 5 cm in 71% of cases. The antrum is the site of predilection (55% of cases), but 21% of patients have multiple sites of disease in the stomach [470, 507].

Secondary involvement is often demonstrated radiologically as large folds corresponding to diffuse lesions. The rare primary forms are solitary or multiple tumors which may cause stenosis or ulceration. Histological confirmation is required to diagnose HD. The diagnosis based solely on radiological appearances is carcinoma (Fig. 7.18).

7.1.2.3 Small Bowel

The small intestine is the second most frequent site of gastrointestinal HD after the stomach, yet fewer than 100 cases were reported before 1976. Sixty-six cases were reviewed in the literature [27, 134, 142, 145, 146, 178, 226, 227, 286, 475, 477, 507, 510, 512, 561]. The general radiological features and frequencies are listed in Tables 7.3 and 7.4. The average patient age is

Table 7.4. Incidence of digestive tract sites of HD

	Esophagus (%)	Stomach (%)	Small bowel (%)	Colon/rectum (%)
Incidence of secondary forms (289)	3.7	11.4	5.2	4.7
Incidence with respect to NHL	Rare	5.6	3.3	Rare
Incidence with respect to other digestive tract sites [71, 289, 662]	2–14.5	35.8–50	24–35	13–27.5

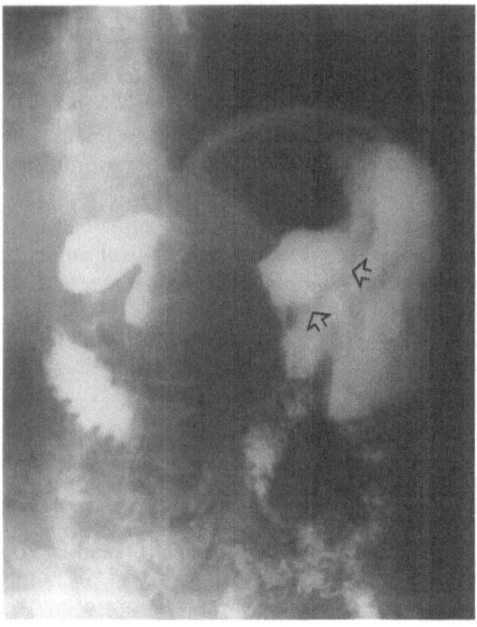

Fig. 7.18. HD of the stomach: ulcerating form *(arrows)*

49 years (range 22–79 years in review cases), and women are affected more often than men. Clinical symptoms, occurring alone or in combination, include abdominal pain (94% of patients), weight loss (59%), vomiting (41%), diarrhea (35.3%), abdominal mass (29.4%), and bleeding (11.7%). In certain cases, intestinal HD can complicate steatorrhea [561] or hemorrhagic rectocolitis [134]. The site of predilection is the jejunum (61.6% of cases), followed by the ileum (23%) and the duodenum (15.4%). Lesions are less than or equal to 5 cm in 78% of cases.

The radiological patterns of HD of the small bowel include infiltrating forms (58%, 43% of which are stenotic), tumoral forms (58%), and ulcerated forms (12%). Complex forms occur in 5% of patients, accompanied by obstruction [134] or signs of intestinal perforation [134, 178]. Sixteen percent of patients have multiple intestinal disease sites. The radiological appearances of tumors and small stenotic infiltrating lesions are usually interpreted as carcinoma before histological confirmation. Arteriography demonstrates small-bowel HD as avascular processes [226].

7.1.2.4 Colon and Rectum

Both primary and secondary HD of the colon and rectum are exceedingly rare, even more so than NHL of these same sites, which is itself infrequent. Only 20 cases affecting the colon were reported before 1970 [353], and fewer than 10 cases involving the rectum were published before 1978 [361]. The general features of colonic and rectal HD were defined on the basis of 20 cases in the literature [44, 154, 209, 256, 261, 353, 359, 507, 653]. Table 7.4 summarizes frequency data. The average patient age is 35 years of age, and male predominance was noted in the review cases. The most common presenting symptoms, in decreasing order of frequency, are weight loss, bleeding, fever, palpable mass, diarrhea, and pain. The cecum is the site of predilection, being affected more often than either the left colon or the rectum. Barium enemas reveal a higher incidence of infiltrating lesions (stenotic or not) than tumoral masses. The rectum is usually affected by nodular forms rather than ulcerating lesions. Diffuse involvement is exceptional [154], and association with an ileal lesion is much less common than in NHL [653]. The rarity of this pathology precludes diagnosis of HD solely from radiological data.

Despite the trophism of malignant lymphomas in the gastrointestinal tract, diagnosis of NHL appears possible using the following radiological criteria:

Large lesions (10 cm or more in over two-thirds of cases, especially in gastric sites)
A general lack of correlation between vague clinical symptoms and marked radiological findings
The frequency of multiple forms, present in nearly one-third of cases (either an association of different forms in a given gastrointestinal segment or involvement of several different segments)
The exceptional nature of stenotic forms owing to the absence of a fibroblastic stroma reaction in NHL

Diagnosis of NHL is especially important, as biopsies are not always conclusive, and patients with gastrointestinal NHL are not always good candidates for surgery. Disease work-ups should include complete studies of the entire digestive tract aimed at detecting any associated tumors, which Zeller found in 20% of cases [675]. By contrast to NHL, both primary and secondary gastrointestinal HD involvement are rare, and always correspond to stage IV lesions. Owing to the absence of a fibroblastic stroma reaction, the radiological findings are often identical to those of carcinoma.

7.2 Malignant Lymphomas of the Spleen, Liver, Biliary Tract, and Pancreas

Whereas the various imaging modalities are all suitable for digestive tract studies, investigation of the solid organs of the abdomen presents specific problems. As the difficulties encountered in the diagnosis of HD and NHL are similar, both patholgies are here treated together for each organ.

7.2.1 Spleen

The spleen is the primary site of NHL or HD in less than 1% of all lymphomas [6]. Non-Hodgkin's etiologies predominate (approximately 75% of all primary splenic lymphomas). Secondary splenic sites of HD are detected in

37.6%–39% of patients during pretherapy work-ups [324, 551] and the autopsy incidence is even higher: 60%–72% of cases [243, 330]. Secondary NHL is a finding in 32.8% of pretherapy work-ups [236].
Nodular NHL is more frequent than diffuse disease [236]. The gross appearance is usually a homogeneous or miliary lesion (73%); solitary and multiple masses are less common (27% for Ahmann [6]). Splenomegaly can cause a 10- to 20-fold increase in the normal weight [153]. This feature is far from constant, however, and is not specific to lymphomas.
Arteriography is the least sensitive and most aggressive radiological technique [26, 182, 320, 528], and is of little diagnostic value. Arteriograms of HD are usually normal; more rarely, they reveal avascular filling defects without hypervascularity (Fig. 7.19). Although hypovascularized nodular lesions predominate in NHL, hypervascularized lesions with heterogeneous neovascularity have also been reported [182].
Radionuclide studies of the spleen can detect splenic enlargement, whether homogeneous or associated with filling defects. The predictive value of splenic involvement is 43% in HD [433].
Ultrasonography appears more sensitive than radionuclide studies for the detection of small nodular lesions. Sonographic patterns include:

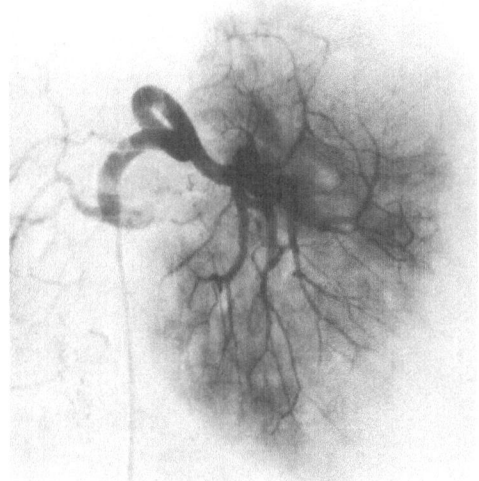

Fig. 7.19. HD of the spleen: nodular pattern demonstrated by angiography

Normal appearance, although this does not rule out lymphoma.

Homogeneous splenomegaly, more or less echogenic than the hepatic parenchyma. This pattern is not specific, however, since similar global modifications in echostructure also occur during vascular congestion and reactive changes (Fig. 7.20).

The existence of hypoechoic and generally multiple nodules 0.5–3 cm in diameter which is less frequent but more suggestive. Even outside of a proven lymphomatous context, this pattern should initially be considered to point to lymphoma (Figs. 7.21 and 7.22).

Solitary tumoral forms of a heterogeneous nature, associating more or less echogenic zones. Splenic hilar adenopathies, often associated with intrasplenic lesions [77, 106, 580].

CT is of limited utility, as its sensitivity has been evaluated at between 17% and 25% [49, 665]. Although CT can easily measure splenic volume, the variable size of the normal spleen makes it difficult to use size as a diagnostic factor. Only nodules 1 cm or more in diameter are currently detectable by CT with or without injection of contrast material [260] (Figs. 7.23–7.25). More recently, intravenous (i.v.) administration of ethiodized oil [Ethiodol oil emulsion 13 (EOE 13)] has been shown to increase the sensitivity of CT to 83% [609] by allowing detection of 5-mm lymphomatous nodules, but use of this technique is still limited to a few institutions.

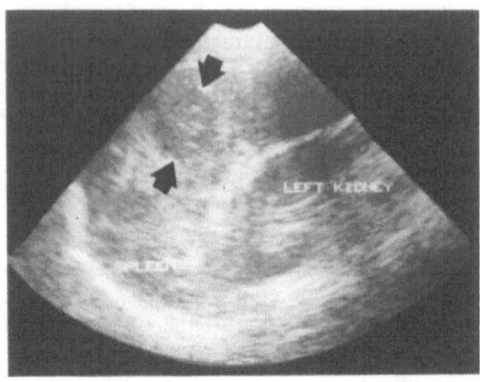

Fig. 7.21. HD: nodular involvement *(arrows)* of the spleen. (Sagittal scan: 36 mm between *arrows*)

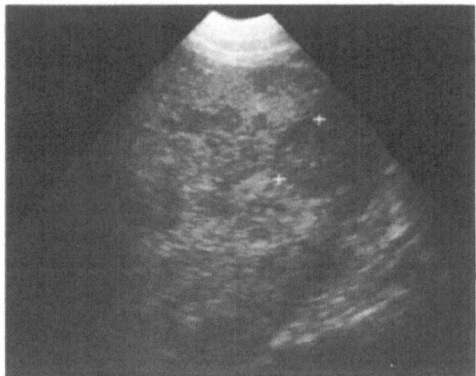

Fig. 7.22. HD: nodular involvement of the spleen. (Sagittal scan: 26 mm between *two crosses*)

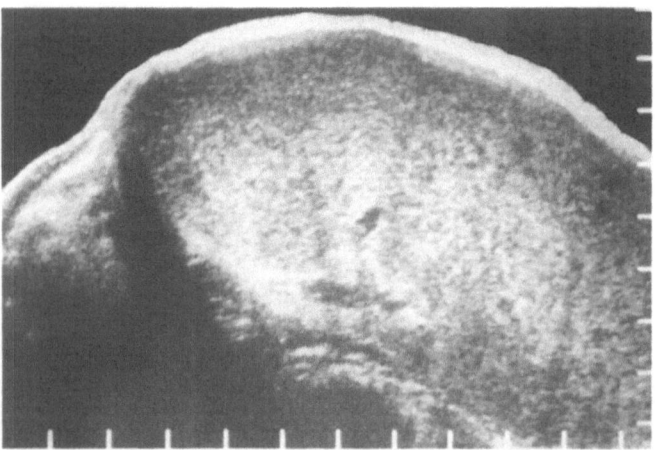

Fig. 7.20. NHL of the spleen: infiltrative pattern. (Transverse scan)

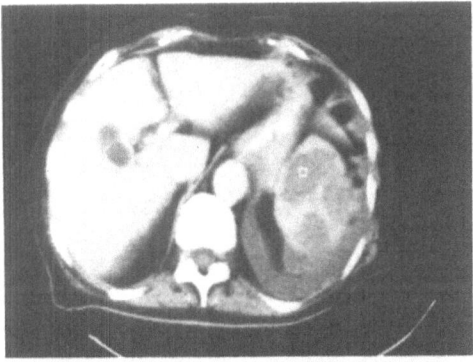

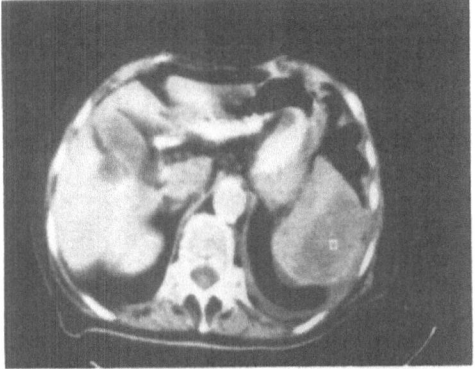

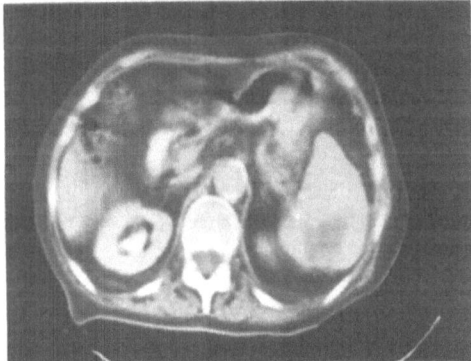

Fig. 7.23. HD: tumoral involvement of the spleen *(square)*

While a certain amount of progress has been made in the investigation of splenic lymphomas, diagnostic accuracy has improved only slightly.

7.2.2 Liver

Like the spleen, the liver has not benefited as much from new imaging modalities as could have been hoped.

Primary involvement is exceptional in HD and accounts for only 0.4% of extranodal NHL [212]. Secondary forms are more frequent: hepatic involvement is noted during pretherapy work-ups for 8%–14% of patients with HD [3, 233, 236, 324]; the autopsy incidence varies from 36% to 74% [233, 243, 330, 341]. The frequency of secondary hepatic NHL ranges from 14% to 27% in pretherapy work-ups [236, 348], and from 50% to 52% in autopsy series [341, 375, 534].

Macroscopically, HD occurs more often as miliary lesions than as solitary or multiple tumors. The lymphocytic forms of NHL tend to be miliary, whereas histiocytic forms are usually nodular or tumoral [341].

Early clinical diagnosis remains difficult, but the more advanced the disease stage, the earlier liver involvement occurs [287]. HD of the liver is always associated with splenic involvement [234, 324], in contrast to NHL [236]. Biological tests are of little value for the detection of NHL [348]. Although both serum 5'-nucleotidase activity and an elevation in alkaline phosphatase are tests with a good sensitivity, their specificity is insufficient for use as determining factors in diagnosing hepatic involvement [3, 38, 157, 314, 348]. Certain authors have advocated liver biopsy as a routine part of NHL work-ups [348], even though this procedure has a certain false-negative rate (18% for Goffinet [236]). Peritoneoscopy also gives a non-negligible number of false-negative results, although multiple biopsies can increase its sensitivity [43, 137, 293].

Of all the available imaging techniques, angiography has the least diagnostic value [110, 131]. Lymphomatous tumors are generally avascular. The angiographic features defined by Chuang [131] include single or multiple masses producing arterial displacement without encasement; sparse tumor vasculature; relative lucency without peripheral dense stain during the hepatogram phase; and absence of arteriovenous shunting, venous laking, or signs of portal obstruction. Less frequently, a hypervascularized mass shows neovascularity [110].

Although radionuclide studies give numerous false-negatives [348], Zornoza [680] has credited this technique with a sensitivity of 71%, a specificity of 81%, and an overall accuracy of 80%. Diffuse enlargement of the liver may or may not be associated with one or more filling de-

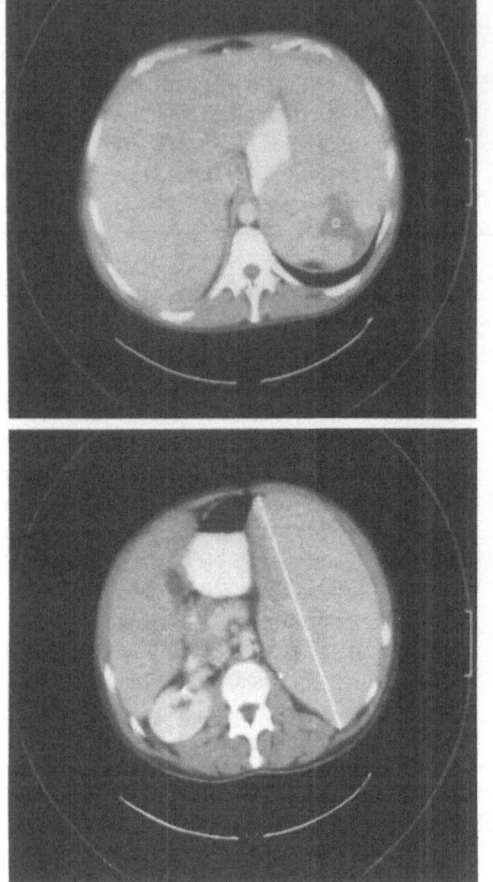

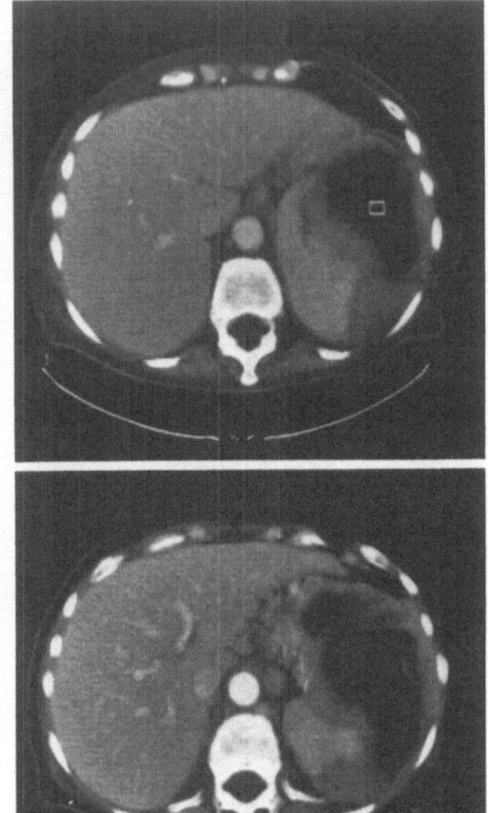

Fig. 7.24. HD: splenomegaly complicated by a small infarction *(square)*. *Bottom: line* connecting *two crosses,* 19.33 cm

Fig. 7.25. NHL: splenic infarction *(square)* which appeared during treatment

fects. False-positives are also possible. The patterns observed are nonspecific, occurring in cirrhosis and hepatitis as well as in lymphomas [433, 680].

For certain authors, the low sensitivity of ultrasound for diagnosis is offset by its value for evaluating response to treatment [232]. As for the spleen, there are several sonographic patterns [77, 104, 202, 232]:

A normal appearance, which does not exclude the possibility of liver involvement.
Diffuse enlargement of the liver (which may or may not be homogeneous).
Hypoechoic, often multiple, nodules (Figs. 7.26 and 7.27).

Anechoic, hyperechoic, or bull's-eye lesions, which are less common [232].
Existence of periportal adenopathies. A search should always be made for such nodes, since they are associated with the above patterns in over one half of cases for Carroll [104].

For Zornoza [680], CT has a sensitivity of 57%, a specificity of 88%, and an overall accuracy of 85%. Intravenous injection of a hydrosoluble contrast material does not improve the sensitivity of this modality for detection of intrahepatic nodules [440] (Fig. 7.28). By contrast, i.v. injection of ethiodized oil increases sensitivity by permitting detection of nodules as small as 5 mm [609, 635].

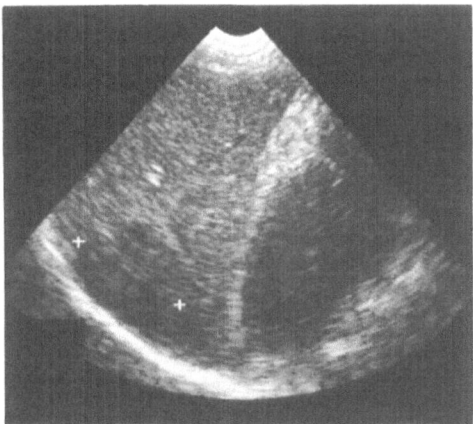

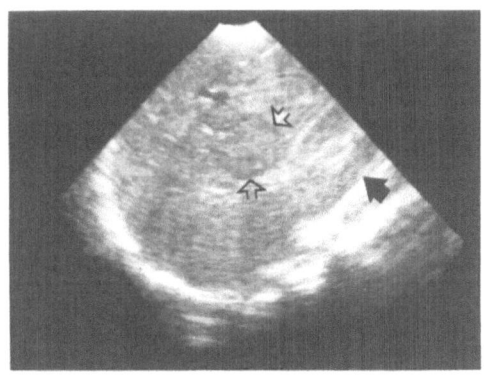

Fig. 7.26. NHL: nodular hypoechoic involvement of the liver. (Sagittal scan: 53 mm between *two crosses*)

Fig. 7.27. HD: nodular hypoechoic involvement of the liver *(white arrows). Black arrow* right kidney

7.2.3 Biliary Tract

Lymphomatous involvement of the biliary tract occurs essentially as the result of disease spread from periportal lymph nodes. Isolated involvement of the bile duct walls is extremely rare. As in HD, primary lesions are exceptional in NHL [461], representing only 0.4% of primary extranodal forms [212].

Secondary involvement is slightly more common, accounting for 0.5% of clinically detected forms in HD and 1.6% in NHL. Autopsy data reveal gallbladder involvement in 2.3% of cases [534, 631].

While histology studies have shown that the biliary tract can be affected by all types of lymphomas [53, 461, 521, 672], involvement is generally the result of nodal invasion of the bile ducts [61, 581, 672]. Concomitant liver involvement occurs in almost all cases [61, 567].

Jaundice, the most frequent clinical symptom, indicates disease of the main duct. However, gallbladder involvement can remain asymptomatic for long periods [461, 567]. Etiological diagnosis is of considerable importance, since radiotherapy has proven extremely effective, making the prognosis for lymphoma much better than that for carcinoma of the pancreas or bile ducts [53].

In secondary forms, the most prevalent, jaundice should suggest periportal node involvement. As a rule, CT and ultrasonography can provide the diagnosis. Radiotherapy can then

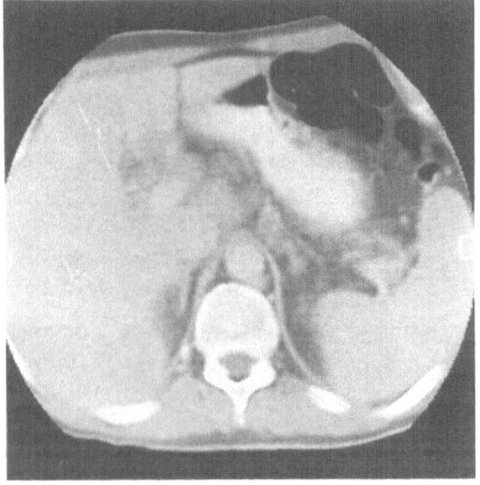

Fig. 7.28. NHL: nodular hypodense involvement of the liver. *Line 1,* 45.2 mm; *Line 2,* 16.6 mm

be given, if necessary after performance of a guided puncture biopsy.

When required, radiological exploration of the biliary tract by endoscopic opacification [521, 567] can reveal compression, infiltration, or localized stenosis of the intrahepatic bile ducts. The extrahepatic bile duct may be dilated above a site of infiltration or extrinsic compression. The gallbladder may or may not be dilated (Fig. 7.29).

The differential diagnoses are sclerosing cholangitis and adenocarcinoma, especially for localized stenosis of the extrahepatic bile duct.

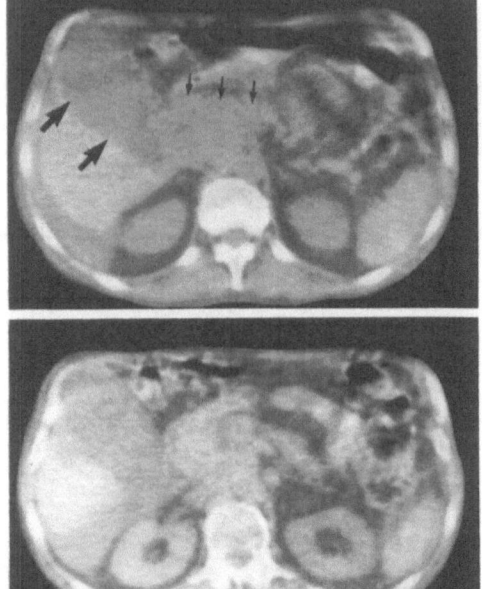

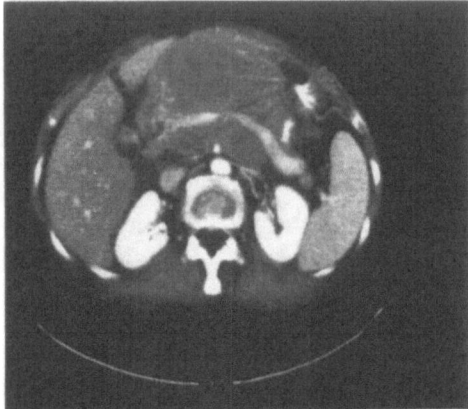

Fig. 7.29. NHL: diffuse infiltration of the head of the pancreas and the biliary tract. (*large arrows*, gallbladder dilatation)

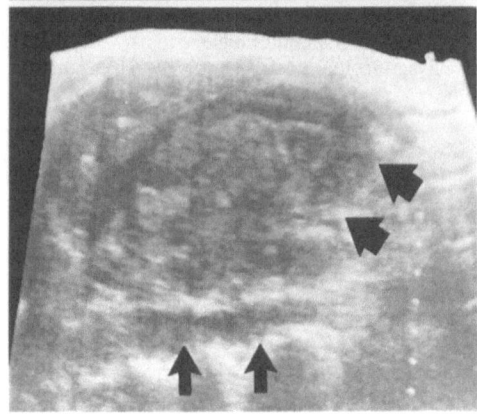

Fig. 7.30. NHL of the pancreas: CT and ultrasound studies. *Large arrows*, tumor; *small arrows*, aorta

7.2.4 Pancreas

Lymphoma accounts for only 0.2% of all malignant tumors of the pancreas [34]. The pancreas is rarely the site of primary HD, and represents only 0.6% of all extranodal NHL sites [212]. Secondary involvement is somewhat more frequent, occurring in 11% of autopsy series for HD [243] and in 29% for NHL [534]. Differential diagnosis from an anaplastic carcinoma is often difficult histologically [4, 672]. Since intraoperative biopsy involves a risk of complications and has a high false-negative rate [4], a formal diagnosis of lymphoma is not always possible. Clinical symptoms and the prognosis (median survival 4 months) are comparable to those of other cancers [34, 672]. Radiological features are also similar to those of pancreatic carcinoma. Ultrasound can visualize glandular enlargement, a hypoechoic gland, and, above all, any peripancreatic nodes [104]. Arteriography is useful for detecting arteriolar infiltration and arterial or venous stasis, generally associated with adenopathies [453,

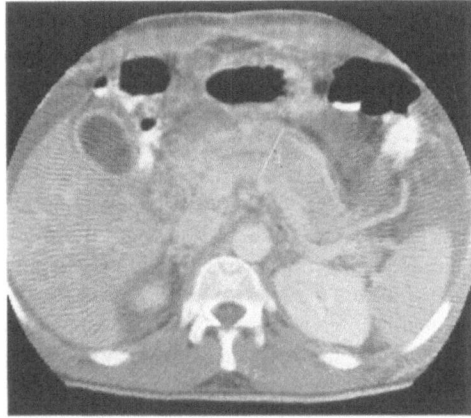

Fig. 7.31. NHL of the pancreas. *Line 1*, 34 mm

625] (Figs. 7.30 and 7.31). Opacification techniques can demonstrate stenosis of the bile ducts or pancreatic ducts, leading to the diagnosis of lymphoma.

While involvement of the biliary tract or pancreas is rare, hepatic and splenic lesions often occur from the outset in lymphomas. Although imaging modalities remain insufficient for diagnosis, future improvements may result from i.v. injection of iodinated emulsions prior to CT and advances in ultrasonographic tissue characterization, which has given promising results in vitro.

8 Lymphomas of the Urinary Tract, the Male Genital System, and the Adrenal Glands

J. DROUILLARD AND J.-N. BRUNETON

Like other extranodal sites of lymphoma, urogenital lesions involve two types of problem related to the circumstances of clinical discovery. Diagnosis is the basic problem for apparently primary forms, whereas discovery of a urogenital lesion during the course of an already recognized or treated lymphoma is an unfavorable prognostic sign.

8.1 Urinary Tract

Specific lymphomatous infiltration of an organ must always be distinguished from the urological consequences of extraurinary lesions such as adenopathies. Non-Hodgkin's lymphomas (NHL) of the urinary tract are more frequent than Hodgkin's disease (HD). Weimar[648], who reported a 6.7% overall incidence of urogenital lesions in his review, cited lesions in 5.8% of patients with HD and in 7.3% of patients with NHL. The kidney was the most common urogenital site of lymphoma in Weimar's study (68% of cases), and renal involvement is the cause of 2.5% of deaths from lymphoma [523].

8.1.1 Kidney

Primary lymphomas of the kidney are extremely rare [267, 423, 579]. Secondary forms, resulting from hematogenous spread or, less often, from contiguous extension of a retroperitoneal lymphoma, are more common [127].
Tumoral proliferation is initially interstitial, displacing but not invading the surrounding healthy tissue. The course of the disease is characterized by progressive compression, then destruction, of normal tissues. Radiological images vary with the type of neoplastic growth:

Lesions with a slow, uniform growth pattern infiltrate the parenchyma and compress the collecting system, but renal contours are preserved.
Multifocal lesions gradually coalesce, and the resulting lymphomatous nodules cause renal enlargement, deformation of the collecting system, and renal insufficiency.
Perirenal lesions can invade the ureter, the vascular pedicle, and the retroperitoneal structures.

The great polymorphism of lymphomatous spread in the kidney explains the diversity of the clinical and radiological pictures [267].

8.1.1.1 General Characteristics

Incidence. Lymphomas are generally cited as the third cause of renal metastases, after primary tumors of the lungs and breast [267, 282]. Renal disease sites have been reported in 38.5%-63% of autopsies [523, 553]. Kidney involvement is less frequent in HD, accounting for 7%-17.5% of autopsy findings [523]. This difference in the frequency of renal lesions between HD and NHL is also reflected in radiological studies [104]. Among types of NHL, diffuse histiocytic forms and Burkitt's lymphoma have the highest frequencies of renal involvement [9, 104, 176, 305].

Macroscopic Appearance. Richmond [523] reported the following frequencies for the various macroscopic forms of lymphoma: multiple nodules, 61%; invasion from perirenal lymphoma, 11%; solitary nodules, 7%; single large tumors, 6%; diffuse infiltration, 6%; and microscopic lesions, 7%. Detection of small multinodular forms has improved through the use of ultrasonography and computed tomography (CT) [127, 423]. Bilateral renal lesions occur in 50%-72% of cases [127, 272, 357, 523].

Clinical and Biological Signs and Symptoms.
The average age of patients at the time of diagnosis of primary or secondary renal lymphomas ranges from 40 to 50 years, although cases have been reported in children [600]. Clinical signs suggestive of renal involvement are infrequent and of late onset, reflecting the long period of interstitital lymphomatous infiltration. Even in the 7.5%–14% of cases in which lymphomatous renal lesions cause clinical manifestations, the resulting symptoms are nonspecific (abdominal pain, deterioration of the patient's general condition, palpable renal mass, and hematuria). Biological anomalies are not specific either. Proteinuria may occur as part of a nephrotic syndrome for which there are three main etiologies: compression of the renal veins by adenopathies, renal amyloidosis, or a paraneoplastic syndrome of immunological origin [536]. Renal insufficiency is a classically late manifestation of the lymphomatous process; however, it occurs in 20%–50% of patients with renal involvement [267, 357, 600].

8.1.1.2 Radiological Exploration

Routine investigative procedures for renal lymphomas include excretory urography, angiography, ultrasonography, and CT.

Excretory Urography (Intravenous Pyelography). Excretory urography has a sensitivity of approximately 60% for renal lymphomas [357]. The major radiological signs [9, 176, 267, 305, 541, 600] include:

Impaired renal function (delayed excretion is more common than nonfunction)
Hydronephrosis, owing to dilatation of the renal calices without dilatation of the renal pelvis (infiltration of the renal sinus), or to dilatation of the excretory cavities (ureteral involvement)
A renal mass, in decreasing order of frequency: a solitary intrarenal mass smaller than 25 mm in diameter; multiple masses in one or both kidneys; a large, nonfunctioning tumoral kidney; or a perirenal mass invading the kidney

Angiography. Despite the polymorphism of renal lymphomas, which produces a wide variety of angiographic findings, several features are

common, although by themselves nondiagnostic [190, 267, 500, 652, 655]:

Stretching of the arteries, usually associated with tumoral hypovascularization; hypervascularization is extremely rare [652]
Palisading of tumor vessels, a suggestive but nonspecific finding [354, 500, 565]
Presence of a capsular artery supplying the tumor (in 54% of cases for Hartman [267] (Fig. 8.1)
Nephrographic irregularities, which can even simulate polycystic disease [258]
Absence of a sharp separation between the tumor and the normal parenchyma.
Opacification of collateral veins involved in renal vein thrombosis, a relatively frequent finding [500]

Renal phlebography has been recommended for the detection of renal vein thrombosis [541], extrinsic encasement causing obstruction [659], and lymphomatous infiltration of the renal veins resulting in kidney insufficiency [171].

Ultrasonography. As for other imaging techniques, no histological correlation has been found between sonographic images and lymphomatous subtypes. The resolution of this

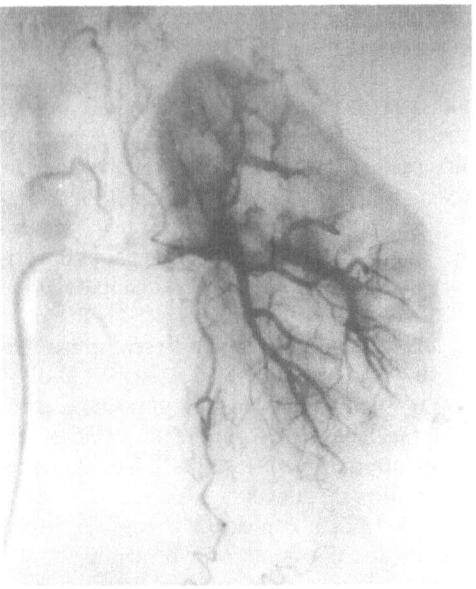

Fig. 8.1. Primary renal lymphoma: tumoral hypovascularization with a peripheral capsular artery

technique in lymphomas allows detection of lesions as small as 0.5 cm [223]. Since most lymphomas have a uniform cellular structure with only slight vascularization, the lesions are generally less echogenic than the adjacent renal parenchyma, although hyperechoic and complex patterns have also been observed [240, 272]. For Carroll [104], most renal lymphomas are uninodular or multinodular hypoechoic focal lesions (Figs. 8.2, 8.3). Diffuse infiltration with or without perirenal involvement is less common. Certain other lymphomatous forms are seen even more seldom. The homogeneity of solitary tumors may be such that they mimic renal cysts, even to the point of producing posterior enhancement [271]. Meticulous ultrasound examination, however, can detect slight irregularities in the posterior wall, and the acoustic enhancement is weaker than with simple cysts [271]. When doubts persist, gallium[67] scans are advisable, since this technique has a sensitivity of 50%–77% for renal lymphomas [574].

Caliceal elongation resulting in disappearance of the normal central renal echoes is another distinct pattern, produced by lesions near the renal sinus. Since such patterns can mimic hydronephrosis, problems may arise in differentiating sinusal lymphomatous infiltration from ureteral compression which is due to adenopathies [202, 249].

In instances of diffuse renal infiltration, the renal parenchyma may appear hypertrophic, with loss of clearly defined contours and no identifiable medulla [16]. Other ultrasonographic features may also be associated with parenchymal lesions. Hydronephrosis, for example, occurs in 22.2%–37.5% of renal lymphomas and corresponds to involvement of the urinary tree [16, 104]. Renal hilar adenopathies are visible in 87.5% of cases [106].

A constellation of several different ultrasonographic findings can be of assistance is diagnosing renal lymphoma, and ultrasound guidance facilitates biopsy for the obtention of histological proof of disease [202]. Ultrasonography is also valuable for assessing the efficacy of therapy, since it can detect changes in lesion size, the disappearance of hypoechoic nodular lesions, and even echostructural modifications, such as the appearance of internal echoes [202, 272].

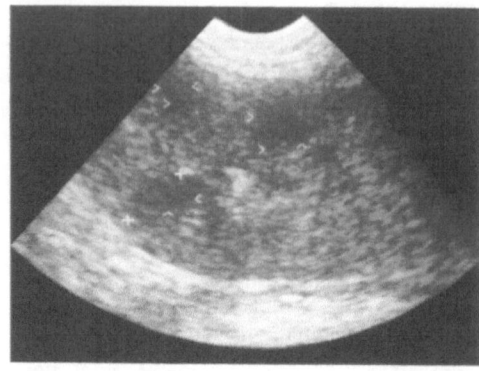

Fig. 8.2. Secondary multinodular lymphoma *(arrowheads)* of the left kidney. (Sagittal scan: 15 mm between the *two crosses*)

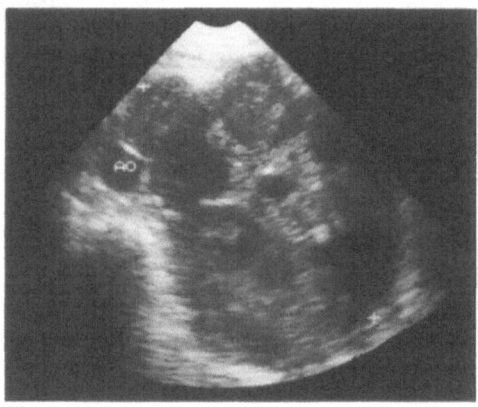

Fig. 8.3. Multinodular disease of the left kidney in angioimmunoblastic lymphadenopathy (AIL). (Transverse scan: 150 mm between the *two crosses*). *AO,* aorta

Computed Tomography. The four morphological forms demonstrated by CT reflect the various anatomical lesion types:

Type I: small solitary nodules (16%–18%) (Fig. 8.4)

Type II: multiple nodules of various sizes (40%–48%) (Figs. 8.5 and 8.6)

Type III: renal infiltration with kidney enlargement (7%–22%) (Fig. 8.7)

Type IV: kidney infiltration by contiguous retroperitoneal adenopathies (20%–29%; [207, 272, 305]); (Fig. 8.8)

Lesions are generally homogeneous and slightly less dense than the normal renal parenchyma [127, 272, 305]; isodense and hyperdense forms are relatively infrequent [352, 456]. In any case, these lesions are always less dense than the healthy parenchyma after the injection of contrast material. Since lymphomatous lesions can be isodense with healthy tissue, systematic use of contrast material is advisable during CT to avoid overlooking renal disease sites.

Other CT-visible abnormalities include:

Presence of retroperitoneal adenopathies (in all cases for Jafri [305])
Thickening of Gerota's fascia and small curvilinear densities in the perirenal space
Hydronephrosis caused by ureteral obstruction of nodal origin

While these features are not suggestive considered alone, an association of several signs

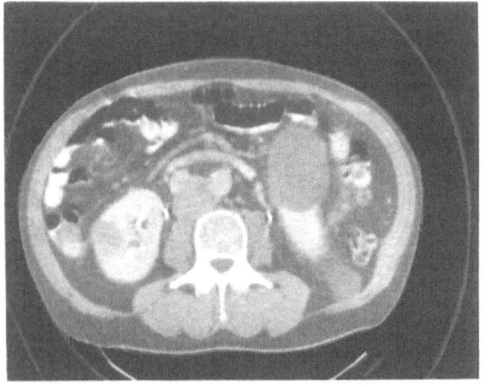

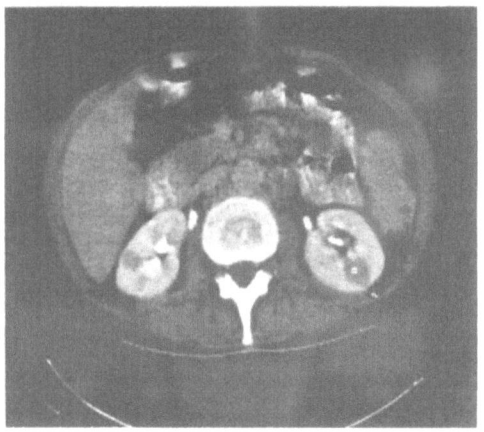

Fig. 8.4 *(above).* Nodular lymphoma of the right kid- ▷ ney with retroperitoneal adenopathies

Fig. 8.5 *(below).* Bilateral multinodular renal lymphoma *(square)*

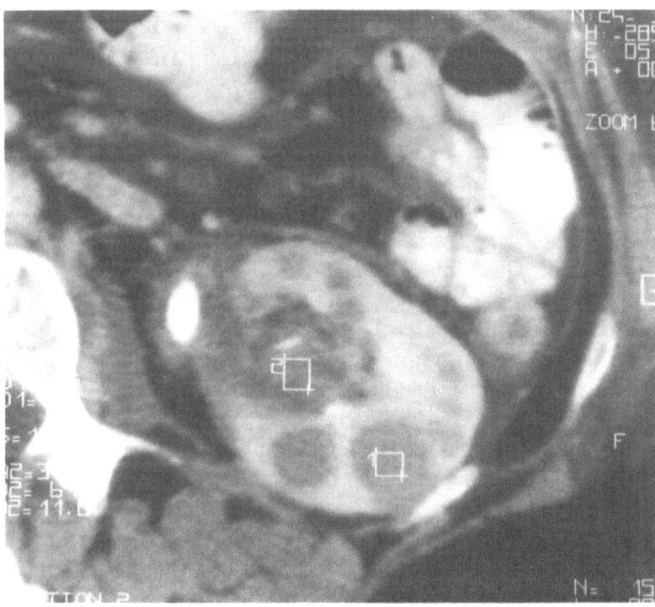

Fig. 8.6. Multinodular lymphoma of the left kidney. *(Square 1,* sinusal fat; *square 2,* nodular, lymphomatous lesion

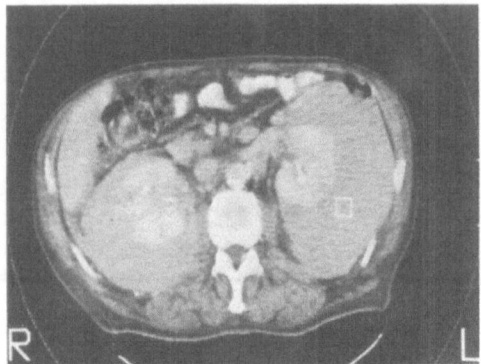

Fig. 8.7. Infiltrating bilateral renal lymphoma *(square)*

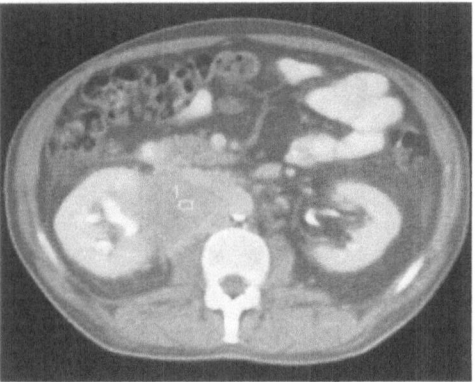

Fig. 8.8. Infiltration of the right renal sinus by lymphomatous adenopathies *(square 1)*

points to lymphoma; diagnosis can be confirmed by fine-needle biopsy.

After chemotherapy, CT scans are helpful in assessing modifications in pre-existent lesions, and especially in small cortical nodules whose largest diameter is under 3 cm. CT facilitates investigation of infiltrating lesions by demonstrating decreases in renal volume, which are occasionally associated with retraction of the renal contour around the lymphomatous zone. Overall, CT is unquestionably the most effective exploratory technique for evaluating the extent of lymphomatous renal involvement before therapy. Likewise, during patient follow-up, CT can assess the need for complementary treatment when radiological images fail to return to normal after chemotherapy.

8.1.1.3 Renal Complications

The renal complications of lymphomas must be carefully distinguished from true renal lymphomas. In addition to complications independent of renal parenchymal lesions, problems may also occur secondary to the treatment of lymphomas.

Renal Complications of Lymphomas. The majority of complications involve retroperitoneal and pelvic adenopathies that can cause secondary ureterohydronephrosis, a finding associated with 4.5%–5.8% of cases [523, 648]. Such stasis can result in lithiasis, infection, or chronic interstitial nephropathy [536]. Renal insufficiency in lymphomas is only rarely the result of lymphomatous infiltration [326]; the most frequent causes are obstruction of the excretory paths, renal vein thrombosis, hypercalcemia-induced nephropathy, and amyloidosis [622].

Treatment-Related Renal Complications. Four types of complication are encountered:

Urinary infections during chemotherapy, occurring in 13% of lymphomas [197].
Acute uric acid nephropathy secondary to administration of cytotoxic agents, which can cause kidney enlargement and nonopacification of the excretory cavities during intravenous pyelography (IVP).
Lithiasis, a classical complication of treatment with allopurinol [16].
Radiation-induced nephritis. Acute forms are rare [380]. Chronic radiation-induced nephritis occurs after approximate doses of 2000 cGy, but the risk is increased by concomitant chemotherapy. Irradiation following therapy with *cis*-platinum requires reduction of the dose to 1500 cGy to avoid radiation-induced complications [222].

8.1.2 Ureter

8.1.2.1 General Characteristics

Lymphomas of the ureter are rare, and care must be taken to differentiate ureteral compression by adenopathies causing superjacent stasis from true forms of ureteral infiltration. The autopsy-determined incidence of such lesions ranges from 7.1% to 9% of all lymphomas [2, 523]. Ureteral lesions are more common in NHL than in HD [632]. Ureteral lesions have been found in up to 16% of autopsies for NHL [553], but true infiltration of the ureter accounts for only 0.86% of autopsy findings [534].

8.1.2.2 Radiological Exploration

CT is indicated for cases of urinary stasis with no obvious etiology, since it can detect adenopathies amenable to puncture biopsy [31, 60]. Indeed, 8%–15% of cases of metastatic nodal involvement have a lymphomatous etiology [135, 240, 392]. Unlike the obstructions caused by other forms of malignancy, these lesions are reversible after treatment (Fig. 8.9).

8.1.3 Bladder

Lymphomas of the bladder are rare, and intrinsic lesions must be distinguished from involvement which is due to lymphomatous pelvic adenopathies. Primary forms are extremely rare in HD; secondary forms account for 4% of autopsy findings [599]. Primary vesical lesions are also rare in NHL (0.13% for Freeman [212]); secondary forms are somewhat more frequent at autopsy (13%) [599].

8.1.3.1 Primary Lymphoma

The fact that only 40 cases of primary bladder lymphoma were reported in the literature until 1971 reflects the rarity of these lesions [20, 522, 646], which unquestionably involve diagnostic problems [406, 590]. The typical patient is a woman aged 60 years of over. Intramural sites predominate, and this explains the problems with diagnosis, since small focal lesions can be hidden by normal or inflammatory mucosa [406]. The radiological images of bladder lymphomas are comparable to those of vesical carcinoma, and certain authors [522, 589] advocate lymphography for the differential diagnosis. In view of the extreme rarity of primary bladder lymphomas, thorough investigatory work-ups are mandatory to detect any concomitant disease sites [656].

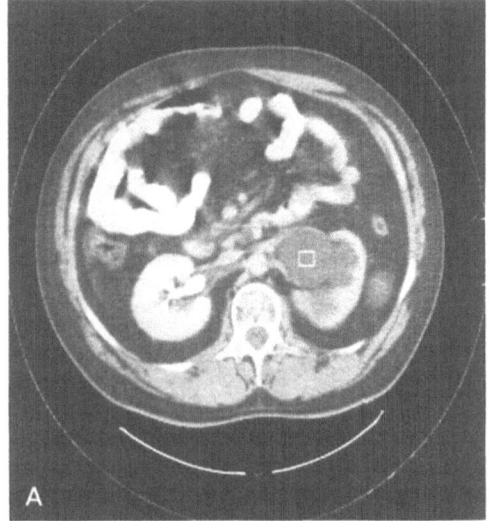

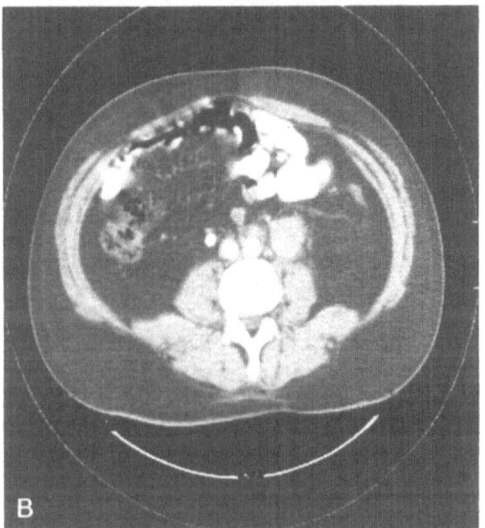

Fig. 8.9. (A) Left renal stasis *(square)* caused by (B) tumoral ureteral obstruction, without any visible adenopathies; surgery revealed ureteral invasion by HD

8.1.3.2 Secondary Lymphoma

Although much more frequent than primary forms, secondary bladder lymphomas cannot always be detected by clinical examination or radiology, since microscopic involvement is approximately 15 times more common than macroscopic lesions [599]. Histological features, and the consequent radiological images, are variable, ranging from nodular lesions confined to the bladder to extrinsic infiltration, or

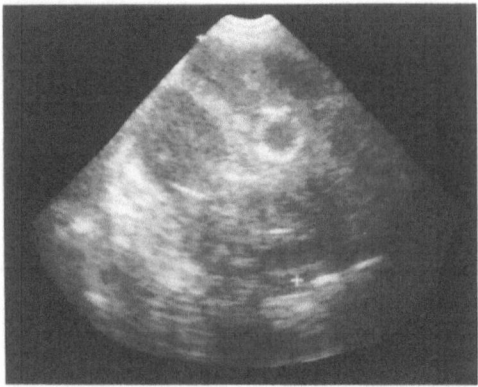

Fig. 8.10. Secondary renal lymphoma 12-cm long; the rounded central image corresponds to the bulb of the bladder probe. (Vertical pelvic scan: 120 mm between the *two crosses*)

combinations of both (Fig. 8.10). There is no correlation with the histological type and no preferential disease site. Diagnosis of bladder lymphoma should be followed by a search for the associated renal and ureteral disease foci present in 94% of cases of NHL and in 55% of cases of HD. Secondary lesions often appear some 18 months before death, announced by clinical signs such as hematuria, dysuria, or infection [646, 656].

As far as diagnosis is concerned, cystoscopy can give erroneous results for intramural forms if the epithelium is intact or there is severe inflammation. The same criticism applies to radiological techniques such as IVP, which has a high false-negative rate because lesions are frequently small. Extrinsic compression caused by adenopathies and ureteral obstruction with hydronephrosis are also possible [656].

Investigation of the bladder wall is facilitated by ultrasonography [659] and CT [183], two techniques which also visualize pelvic and retroperitoneal nodes. Modifications resulting from treatment, and irradiation in particular, can result in radiological images of bladder wall thickening with trabeculation and loss of overall bladder capacity owing to elevation of the pelvic floor. These features are not specific, however, and can be hard to distinguish from lymphomatous recurrence [247]. Cystitis-related lesions resulting from treatment with cyclophosphamide can also prove difficult to differentiate from recurrent disease.

8.2 Male Genital System

While both the prostate and the testis can be affected by primary lymphoma, most lesions occur as part of the generalization of a lymphoma.

8.2.1 Prostate

Primary lymphoma of the prostate is exceptional [259], accounting for only 0.2% of Freeman's series [212]. Autopsy data for secondary forms indicate prostatic involvement in up to 23% of cases [523]. Average patient age is 60 years. The clinical picture usually suggests benign prostatic hypertrophy [168]. The banality of presenting symptoms for both primary and secondary lesions is reflected in the nonspecific nature of radiological findings, whether obtained by ultrasonography or IVP. In our experience, ultrasound visualizes solid, heterogeneous masses lacking even the only very slightly echoic or anechoic structure of lymphomatous nodes (Figs. 8.11 and 8.12).

8.2.2 Testis

The testis, like the rest of the urogenital tract, is rarely the site of primary or secondary HD. Gowing [243] reported only a single case of testicular lymphoma in his series of 130 autopsies for HD. NHL accounts for 4%-7.5% of all malignant testicular tumors [427, 519]. Estimates of testicular NHL vary from 0.2% to 1.6% [212, 606, 648]; the incidence rises to 10% for secondary lesions [427].

Certain anatomical particularities warrant mention. Firstly, owing to the difficulty in diagnosing a primary lymphoma, only a thorough disease extension work-up can determine whether an apparently focal lesion actually is part of a disseminated process from the outset [340, 519]. For Tepperman [606], primary testicular lymphoma, which can be cured by orchidectomy alone, remains a rare entity representing less than 11% of testicular lesions. Diffuse histiocytic forms are the most commonly encountered histological type. Bilateral lesions have been reported in 16%-23% of cases [519, 524, 623], and half of all patients with a bilateral testicular tumor have lymphoma [340].

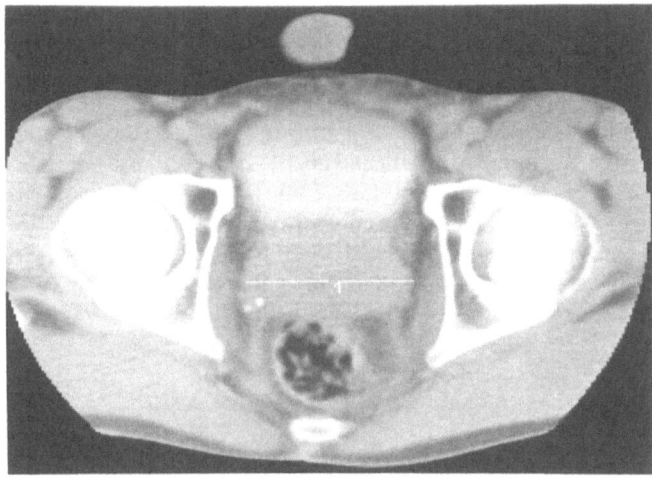

Fig. 8.11. Sonographically heterogeneous prostatic lymphoma. *Line 1,* 68.5 mm

Age is a fundamental clinical factor. The average age of 59 years at onset [519, 606, 623] is considerably greater than the average for teratomas (31 years) or seminomas (40 years). However, cases have also been reported in children [427]. Clinical features include an occasionally bilateral testicular mass; although the tumor may appear solitary, the course of the disease can include distant spread to the skin, nasopharynx, bone marrow, and brain [340, 606].

Ultrasonography is the imaging procedure of choice, at least for investigation of focal lesions [504]. Testicular tumors (Fig. 8.13) are demonstrated sonographically as well-delineated, weakly echogenic zones occasionally associated with a hydrocele, thickening of the scrotal skin, or enlargement of the epididymis. Ultrasound is thus indicated for the exploration of enlarged testes, since a hypoechoic intratesticular mass is suggestive of lymphoma in patients over 50 years of age, and for the surveillance of the remaining testis after unilateral castration. Both CT and ultrasonography are indicated for the work-up of testicular lymphomas, since these lesions are generally only the initial extranodal site of a generalized lymphoma.

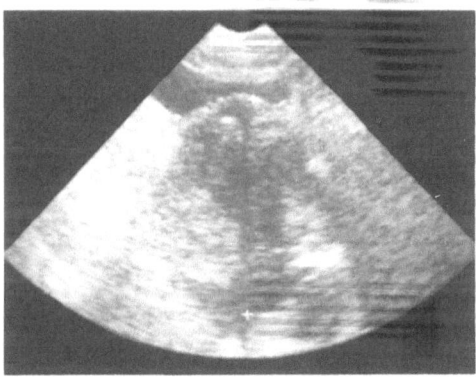

Fig. 8.12. Primary prostatic lymphoma (87 mm between the *two crosses*)

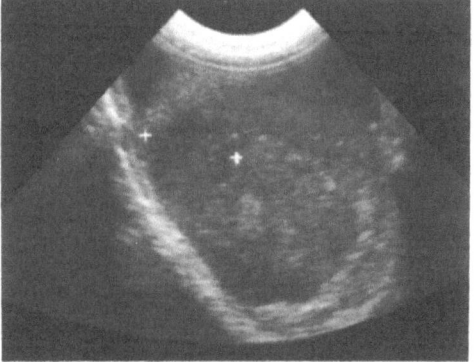

Fig. 8.13. Testicular lymphoma with a solid, multinodular echostructure (15 mm between the *two crosses*)

8.3 Adrenal Glands

Generally clinically asymptomatic, both unilateral and bilateral adrenal gland lymphomas are relatively infrequent [22], accounting for 14.5% of autopsy findings for HD and 20.5%–29% of autopsy findings for NHL [523, 534]. The frequency of lymphoma as the etiology of adrenal lesions is diversely appreciated. For Siekavizza [578], lymphoma is the second cause of adrenal metastases after breast cancer and before lung cancer. By contrast, for Jafri [306], lymphoma represents only 0.64% of CT-detected adrenal lesions. CT is the technique of choice for radiological exploration of the adrenal glands. Adrenal lymphomas are visualized as rounded or oval, uni- or bilateral lesions that are often associated with retroperitoneal adenopathies (85% of cases) and renal disease sites (43% of cases); a systematic search for these related sites of involvement is thus advisable [306] (Fig. 8.14).

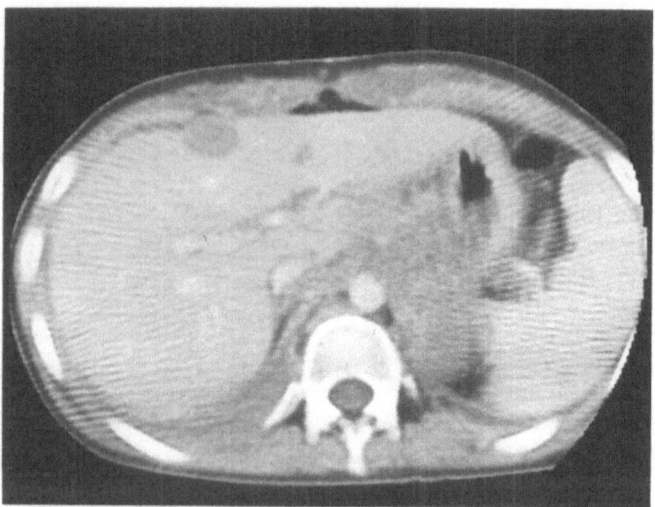

Fig. 8.14. Lymphomatous involvement of the left adrenal gland and liver

9 Gynecological Lymphomas

D. AUBANEL AND J.-N. BRUNETON

Gynecological lymphomas are rare, with non-Hodgkin's lymphomas (NHL) being only slightly more common than Hodgkin's disease (HD). Primary gynecological lesions account for only 2.2% of all extranodal NHL [212]. The majority of gynecological lymphomas occur in the breast; the ovaries and uterus are affected much less frequently.

9.1 Breast

Both primary and secondary lymphomas of the breast are rare. Histologically, most cases concern NHL. Various literature reviews cited some 175 cases in 1981 [156, 535, 559], only 6.1% of which concerned HD [535]; 93.9% dealt with NHL. Depending on the author, primary NHL of the breast represents 0.12%–0.53% of all malignant breast tumors [279, 407, 603, 658] and 10% of all mammary sarcomas [658]. Secondary mammary lesions are extremely rare for both HD (0.8% of autopsy findings for Gowing [243] and for NHL (less than 1% for Rosenberg [534] and Ti [612]).

Histocytic forms are the most prevalent histological type of NHL. Needle aspiration and cytology rarely permit diagnosis, and lymphoma is recognized only after extemporaneous intraoperative examination. Macroscopically, NHL presents as nodular lesions similar in appearance to medullary or anaplastic carcinomas, but quite different from spiculated adenocarcinomas. HD generally occurs as infiltrating lesions whose characteristics are less typical in mammary sites than in nodal locations.

Female predominance is marked; masculine mammary affections of lymphomatous origin remain exceptional [638]. Primary forms essentially affect women of around 60 years of age, although bilateral lesions have been reported in 30-year-old women and post partum [494]. The right breast is involved more often than the left breast, the sites of predilection being the upper outer quadrant and the areola. The lesion generally consists of a hard nodule with an average diameter of 3 cm. Multiple palpable tumors are present in 20% of cases, and half of all patients have palpable axillary nodes.

Secondary forms are encountered in patients of all ages. Edematous forms suggestive of mastitis are seen in 60% of cases. Breast inflammation of this type may be caused either by lymphedema secondary to obstruction of a lymph node, or by true lymphomatous infiltration. Locoregional adenopathies are extremely common.

The prognosis for primary lesions varies greatly from one author to another, ranging from 0 to 64% at 5 years and from 0 to 36% at 10 years [156, 212, 417]. Average survival for secondary forms is even shorter: less than 1 year [417] for both NHL and HD.

Primary and secondary mammary lymphomas demonstrate three main mammographic patterns [251, 417, 430, 638]:

Large, Solitary Opacifications. These dense, homogeneous, and occasionally multilobulated masses measure an average of 3 cm in diameter (range 1.5–6 cm). In young women with dense breasts, the margins can be irregular and ill defined. The adjacent tissue is often displaced, and the tumor is surrounded by a lower-density halo [251]. Skin thickening is rare, except in cases of superficial tumors. Except for medullary and mucinous carcinomas, which have the same appearance, other types of cancer can be ruled out radiologically, owing to the habitual absence of spiculations, microcalcifications, and skin thickening. Cysts can be excluded, as lymphomatous lesions are solid, and the possibility of adenofibroma is generally rejected, as mammary lymphomas are characterized by

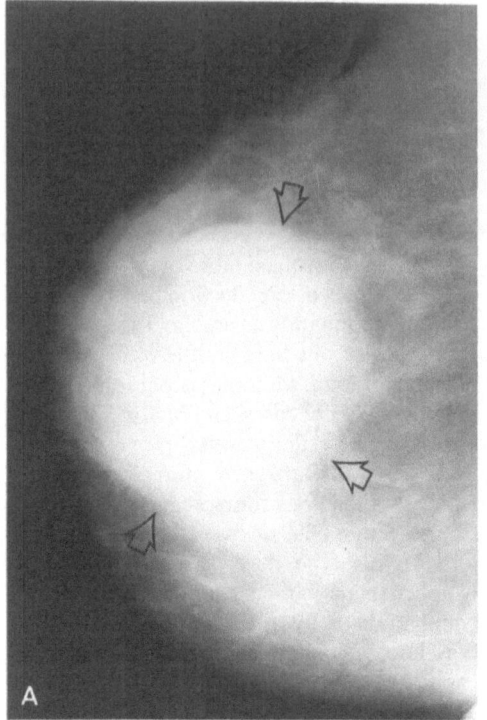

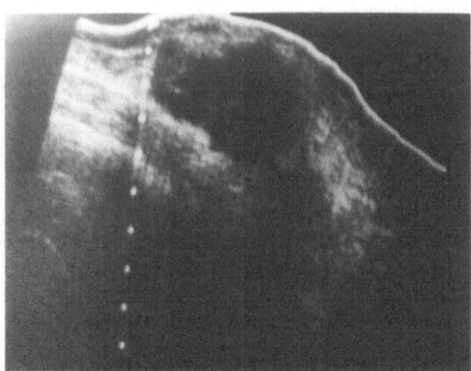

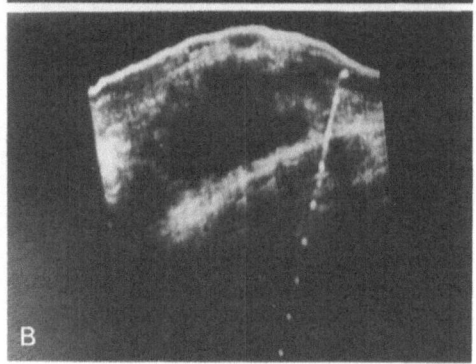

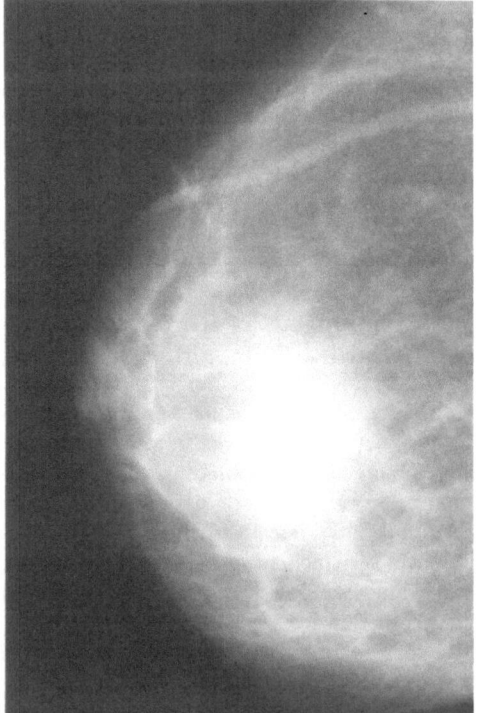

△ **Fig. 9.1 A, B** *(above).* Lymphoma of the right breast.
A Mammogram; **B** sonogram

◁ **Fig. 9.2** *(lower left).* Primary lymphoma of the breast

rapid growth. Primary lymphomas are generally demonstrated as solitary, rounded opacifications (Figs. 9.1–9.3).

Multiple Nodular Opacifications. Although confusion is possible with fibrocystic mastosis,
these nodules are solid, and when located close
together form a conglomerate suggestive of
lymphoma. Glandular edema is more frequently associated with this form than with solitary
nodular lesions. Multiple nodules are encountered essentially with primary lymphomas
(Fig. 9.4).

Inflammatory Disease. Increased density of either the entire breast or at least one half is
caused by inflammatory disease. Diffuse skin
thickening is especially marked in the para-are-
olar region, and the only factor against a diagnosis of carcinomatous mastitis is the absence

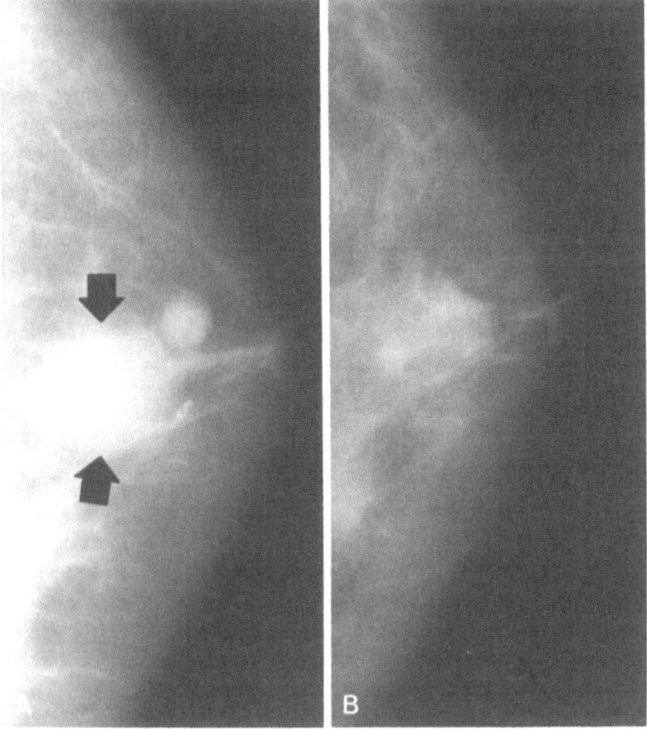

Fig. 9.3 A, B. Lymphoma of the right breast. **A** Before and **B** 2 months after radiotherapy

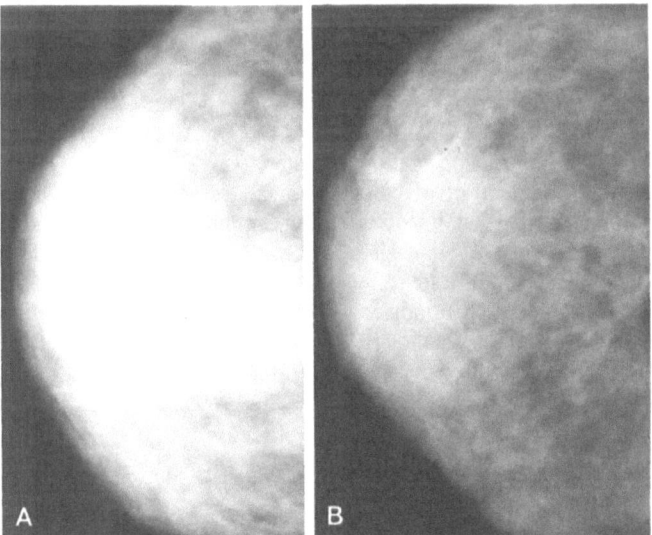

Fig. 9.4 A, B. Multinodular lymphoma. **A** Before and **B** 2 months after radiotherapy

of microcalcifications. This pattern is observed predominantly in secondary lymphomas.

As reported by Viganotti [638], the only author to have studied lymphomas using thermography, hyperthermia is discrete (2°-3 °C), and the hyperthermal surface of thermographically detected forms is identical in size to that shown on the radiological image. While these thermographic criteria are not specific for malignancy, their presence in connection with radiological images suggesting benign lesions should raise the suspicion of a malignant process.

9.2 Ovary

Both primary and secondary ovarian lymphomas are extremely rare. Non-Hodgkin's lesions are by far the most prevalent primary form, representing 92.5%-95% of all cases [129, 538]. However, primary ovarian lymphomas account for only 0.2% of all lymphomas [129] and only 0.5% of all extranodal primary NHL [212]. Ovarian involvement is slightly more common in generalized disease and with secondary forms: ovarian lesions have been reported in 5.1%-9.1% of autopsies for HD [276, 391] and in 9.1%-40% of autopsies for secondary NHL. The highest incidence for autopsy findings is the 58.3% found by O'Conor [473] in a population of African children. Overall, secondary lesions are six times more frequent than primary forms [455].

Macroscopically, ovarian lesions are solid, encapsulated masses which tend to be homogeneous rather than cystic; bilateral involvement occurs in 43%-55% of cases [538, 663]. Nodular histiocytic forms are the most prevalent histological type in NHL [129, 147, 538]; the differential diagnosis is a granulosa cell tumor or a dysgerminoma. Clinical symptoms include pelvic pain and a palpable mass. Primary lymphoma can be discovered during pregnancy. Se-venteen percent of patients have ascites. The prognosis for ovarian NHL is less favorable than for other sites: average survival is only 11 months for stage I disease and 7 months for all other stages considered together [129].

No radiological studies have been published on ovarian lymphoma. In our experience, these lesions tend to be solid, heterogeneous masses with few or no cystlike zones. Lesion contours appear multilobulated on sonograms, and the usual diagnosis is an ovarian tumor of probably malignant origin (Fig. 9.5).

9.3 Uterus

The incidence of lymphomas of the uterus is comparable to that of ovarian lymphomas. Whitaker [151] found only 22 cases in his literature review covering 21 years. NHL predominates (80.8%). Primary uterine sites of NHL account for approximately 0.5% of all extranodal NHL [212]. Primary Hodgkin's lesions are rare [37, 651].

Autopsy data for both HD and NHL confirm the rarity of uterine involvement, even during generalized disease: the autopsy incidence is only 6.8% in NHL [313, 666], and varies from 0.8% to 9.1% in HD [243, 391].

When a cervical lesion is detected, there is a risk that investigation will be limited to cytologic study, giving a consequent diagnosis of only chronic inflammatory lymphocytic infiltrate [65]. Clinical detection of an enlarged corpus uteri generally results in a diagnosis of fibroma. Focal lesions are often diagnosed as polyps [666], while the clinical diagnosis for cervical lesions (Fig. 9.6) is usually cancer [97].

Long periods of survival, ranging from 8 to 24 years [666], have been reported for primary uterine NHL. No radiological studies were found in the literature.

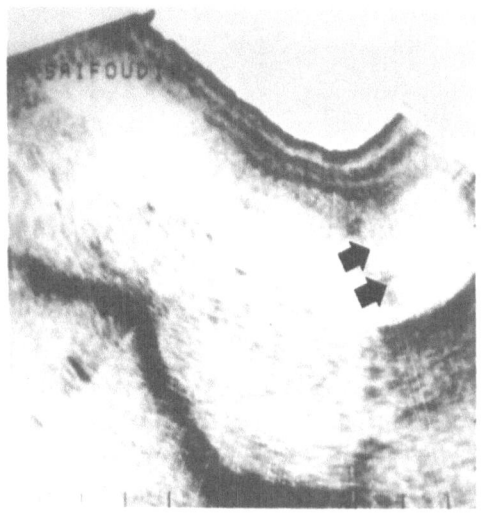

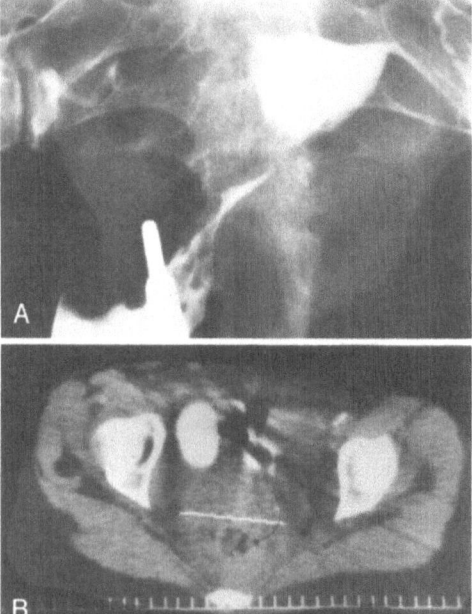

Fig. 9.5. Sonogram of a solid ovarian lymphoma (*arrows;* posterior limits of the nearly empty bladder)

Fig. 9.6 A, B. Lymphoma invading the endocervix. **A** Hysterogram and **B** CT scan

10 Lymphomas of Bone

D. VANEL

10.1 Hodgkin's Disease

10.1.1 Mechanism of Appearance

Hodgkin's disease (HD) of bone can arise by two different mechanisms. In the majority of cases, the initial disease focus is nodal; the osseous lesions are contiguous and reflect progressive invasion of the bone by the nodal mass (Fig. 10.1). The most frequent bone sites (the spine, the pelvis, and the sternum) are thus those in the proximity of the most commonly affected lymph nodes. Less frequently, bone involvement occurs as the result of hematogenous spread, in the same manner as metastasis to bone (Fig. 10.2). Differentiation of the two mechanisms is essential, since their staging and prognosis differ.

10.1.2 Incidence

Frequency data based on skeletal radiography surveys differ greatly from those of autopsy series. Radiologically demonstrable bone lesions are seen in approximately 15% of patients during life [35]. The much higher incidence in autopsies (50%–100%) reflects the fact that smaller lesions are found; in addition, most patients die with terminal disease diffusion.

Diagnostic bone lesions are much rarer, the general consensus being around 2% in the various series [62, 126, 583, 597]. In the H5 study conducted by the European Organization for Research on Treatment of Cancer (EORTC) from 1977 to 1982, only 4 cases of initial osseous disease resulting from contiguous spread were seen in 188 stage I patients, and only 7 cases were observed in 303 stage II patients. Of the 139 new patients examined at the Gustave-Roussy Institute (Villejuif, France) from

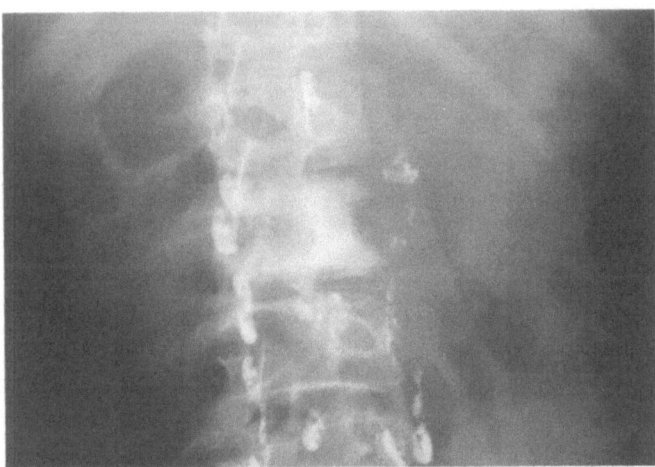

Fig. 10.1. Girl aged 10 years. Pain in the left leg with motion and back pain. The sedimentation rate is elevated. The chest radiograph reveals left hilar adenopathy. Lymphography demonstrates a pathologic process in the left lumbo-aortic region. The body of L 3 is sclerotic, with the distinctive pattern of destruction corresponding to contiguous spread from a nodal mass

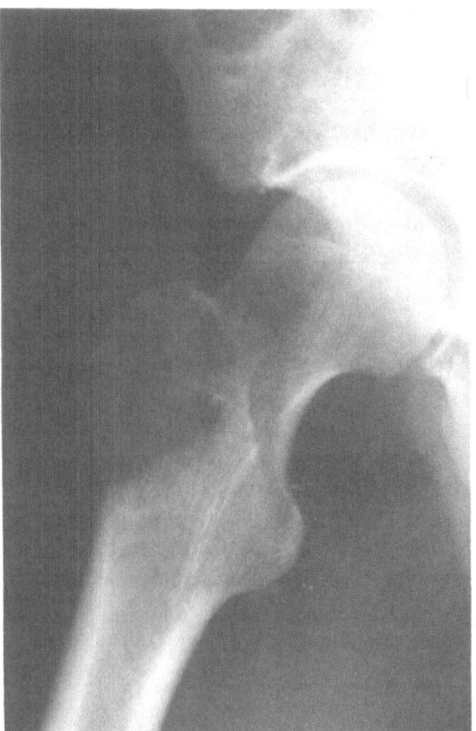

Fig. 10.2. Man with HD. Onset of pain in the lower right extremity: poorly delimited, apophyseal-metaphyseal lytic tumor that has partially destroyed the cortical bone

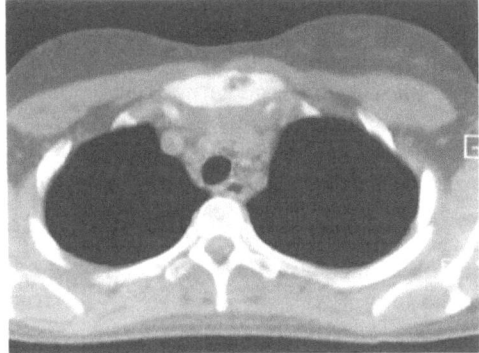

Fig. 10.3. Woman aged 26 years. Sternal swelling led to the discovery of multiple adenopathies (nodular sclerosing HD). CT demonstrates a pre- and retrosternal mass with partial sternal osteolysis

1970 to 1979, 7 had initial bone involvement which was not due to contiguous extension (stage IV). The sites of predilection, in decreasing order of frequency, are the spine (especially the lumbar spine), pelvis, sternum, ribs, shoulder girdle, femurs, and skull. In fact, any bone can be affected.

10.1.3 Clinical Features

The age of patients with bone involvement is the same as that of the general HD population (predominance between 20 and 40 years). Both sexes are equally affected. Presenting symptoms include pain, swelling, and, less often, spinal cord compression. Pain, the most common initial manifestation, may be moderate before becoming severe. One particularity is the fact that pain may be brought on or aggravated by the consumption of alcohol, but this almost path-

ognomonic feature is rare. Pain generally precedes radiological signs by several months.

Osseous swelling depends on the bone affected. The most frequent location is the sternum, and sternal swelling is a classic sign (Fig. 10.3). Swelling of other bones is less common, and spontaneous fracture and vertebral collapse are very rare.

Whether the result of vertebral collapse or, more often, of lymphogranulomatous extension along a nerve root, involvement of the spinal cord or nerve roots seldom leads to diagnosis. Hypertrophic pulmonary osteoarthropathy is an exceptional diagnostic finding. and generally indicates diffuse thoracic involvement.

10.1.4 Radiographic Appearance

10.1.4.1 Radiological Patterns

Bone investigations are not systematic, nor are radionuclide bone scans or complete skeletal surveys. Specific studies are performed as a function of clinical findings. During the course of the disease, multiple sites are the rule (two-thirds of cases); the radiological appearance is often heterogeneous. By contrast, pathognomonic lesions are solitary in approximately two-thirds of cases.

Three radiological patterns of bone destruction have been defined.

Lytic Forms. By far the most prevalent, lytic forms occur as rather poorly defined lucencies, usually with moth-eaten or permeative margins. Invasion by a nodal mass and primary bone lymphomas produce different appearances. Cortical destruction is frequent in primary bone lymphomas, and both lamellated periosteal reaction and Codman's triangle may occur. Perpendicular periosteal new bone formation is much rarer. As these signs correspond to primary bone involvement, they can be used to rule out invasion by a nodal mass.

Contiguous spread from a nodal mass (Fig. 10.1) can cause a purely reactive, solitary lamellated periosteal reaction (even though the nodes may not yet have invaded the bone), which is followed by osteolysis from the outside of the bone to the inside, without periosteal reaction opposite the soft-tissue lesion (although peripheral periosteal involvement is possible) or perpendicular periosteal reaction. Involvement of the neighboring joints is possible but infrequent, and results from direct invasion by tumoral tissue (Fig. 10.4).

Sclerotic Forms. Mainly encountered in the lumbar spine, sclerotic forms correspond to reaction of the normal bone rather than to tumoral osteogenesis. The classic appearance is the "ivory vertebra." Sclerotic change of this type can regress after treatment [244]. Although uninvolved at first, the disks can be affected in the later stages of advanced disease. Multiple sclerotic foci with irregular contours occur in rare instances.

Mixed Lytic and Sclerotic Forms (Fig. 10.5). The radiological appearance has been linked to the histological type, and can also be of prognostic value [67]. Histological types with a good prognosis (lymphocyte predominance, nodular sclerosis) are associated with bone lesions in only 11% of cases, with sclerotic forms accounting for the great majority. By contrast, bone involvement is reported in 64% of patients with histological types of poor prognosis (mixed cellularity, lymphocyte depletion); the lesions in

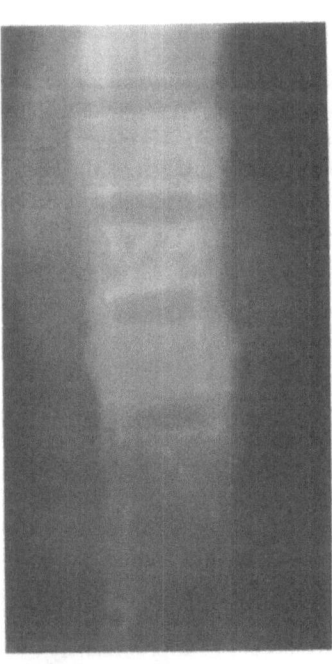

Fig. 10.4. Boy aged 13 years with nodular sclerosing HD; mixed tumor of the dorsal spine with vertebral collapse

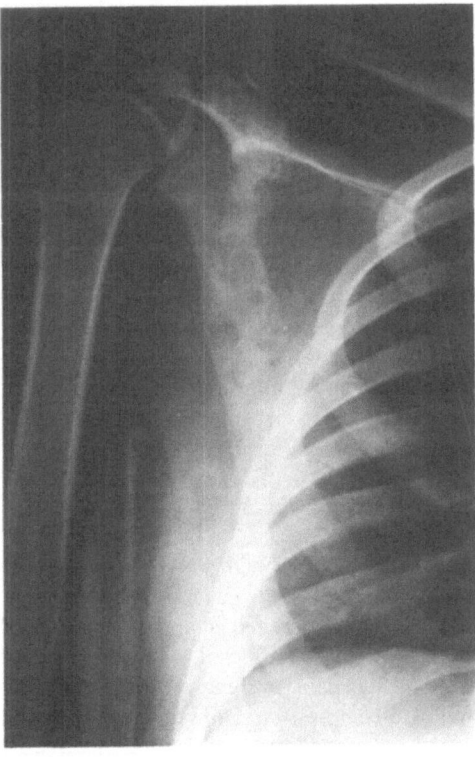

Fig. 10.5. Girl aged 14 years with pain on the right side. Film of the scapula reveals a mixed lytic and sclerotic tumor in the body of the scapula

these cases tend to be purely lytic forms exhibiting permeative bone destruction. Analysis of radiologically demonstrable lesions thus provides an indication as to prognosis: purely lytic lesions, and bone lesions in general, carry a poor prognosis. Medullary involvement demonstrated by bone biopsy is much more common in mixed cellularity disease [184, 531].

10.1.4.2 Anatomical Distribution of Radiological Features

Spine. An "ivory vertebra" is highly suggestive, but not pathognomonic. Striations suggestive of an angioma, caused by reactive hypertrophy of the remaining trabeculae, are much rarer. Anterior or anterolateral erosion of a vertebral body indicates invasion by a soft-tissue mass (Fig. 10.1). This appearance is also highly suggestive of HD, but again is not pathognomonic. It can be seen in connection with any soft-tissue tumor, and especially the nodal metastases of solid tumors (relapses of cervix uteri cancers, for example). Generally, only one or a few vertebrae are involved; the disks are preserved. Vertebral collapse occurs late in the course of the disease. A fusiform image is indicative of adenopathies. Bone invasion by soft-tissue masses can be demonstrated by lymphography (Fig. 10.6) or, even better, by CT. Lesions of the posterior vertebral arch may be lytic or sclerotic and involve the pedicles, the articular processes, or the transverse processes (Fig. 10.7).

Sternum. Sternal lesions [676] occur mainly in the manubrium as lytic lucent defects, often with sharp contours. Multiple lucencies are frequent, reflecting sternal invasion by multiple adenopathies. Lateral erosion is less common. The soft-tissue mass is usually retrosternal, but may also be pre- or laterosternal (Fig. 10.3).

Ribs. Costal involvement can occur as lysis of the extremity of a rib, which is often associated with a sternal or spinal lesion (Fig. 10.7); local expansion or "ballooning" of a costal arch, with thinning of the cortical bone; or bone destruction with longitudinal periosteal reaction.

Pelvis. Pelvic lesions are often mixed, with the osteosclerosis reflecting bone reaction to invasion by pelvic nodes.

Long Bones. Metaphyseal lesions predominate, although disease can occur in diaphyseal sites. Epiphyseal and articular involvement are rare (Fig. 10.7).

10.1.5 Differential Diagnosis

Bone lesions generally appear during the course of recognized HD. Lesions of the femoral and humeral heads can simulate osteonecrosis (Fig. 10.8), and the patient's history must therefore be consulted as to any previous corticosteroid therapy, radiotherapy, or chemotherapy [175, 280, 436]. The role of relevant associated trauma has also recently been emphasized. The differential diagnosis for diagnostic lesions depends on the site. Histiocytosis and benign tumors, for example, are rarely envisaged for spinal lesions. Infection can be entertained when involvement is confined to a vertebra and does not affect the disks. The most difficult problem is differentiation from bone metastases. Radiation-induced bone sarcomas have been described, but are very rare [585].

10.1.6 Classification of Bone Involvement

Lesions resulting from contiguous spread and hematogenous dissemination are classed differently. With contiguous spread, the bone is affected from the outside in; there is no periosteal reaction at the point of contact with the center of the soft-tissue tumor and no perpendicular periosteal reaction. CT is extremely useful for direct evaluation of tumor size. The Ann Arbor classification considers bone involvement resulting from contiguous spread to be extranodal, and patients can be staged I E or II E. Survival at 4 years for the 2% of patients with initial bone lesions resulting from contiguous spread seen at the Gustave-Roussy Institute was 0.92 ± 0.02. These lesions thus do not modify the course of the disease or the prognosis. By contrast, lesions resulting from hematogenous dissemination are classed stage IV from the outset. Literature evaluations of the prognosis for patients with bone involvement by HD vary considerably. In several of the older series, patients with bone lesions had better survival rates than those without, but this prob-

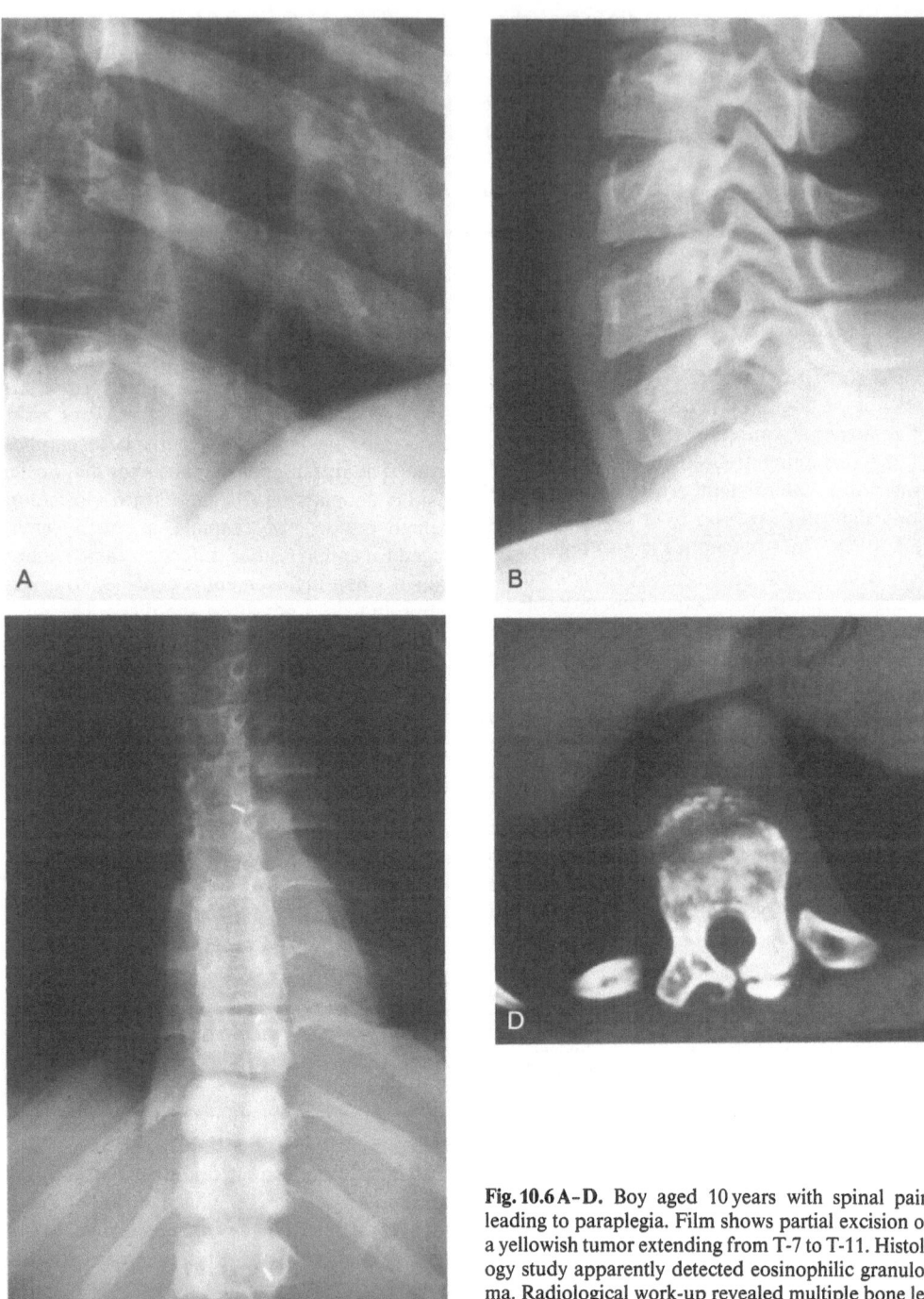

Fig. 10.6 A–D. Boy aged 10 years with spinal pain leading to paraplegia. Film shows partial excision of a yellowish tumor extending from T-7 to T-11. Histology study apparently detected eosinophilic granuloma. Radiological work-up revealed multiple bone lesions in addition to a T-1 lesion. Note **A** the osteolysis of the posterior arch of the ninth left rib and the fusiform vertebra, and **B** the mixed lytic and sclerotic lesion of the body of C 7. The fusiform, paravertebral lesion gradually grew, and sclerotic lesions occurred in T-10 and T-11 (**C, D**). Biopsy of a left axillary node corrected the diagnosis: HD

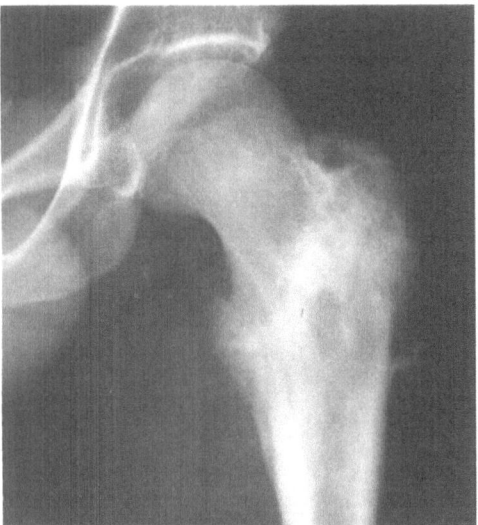

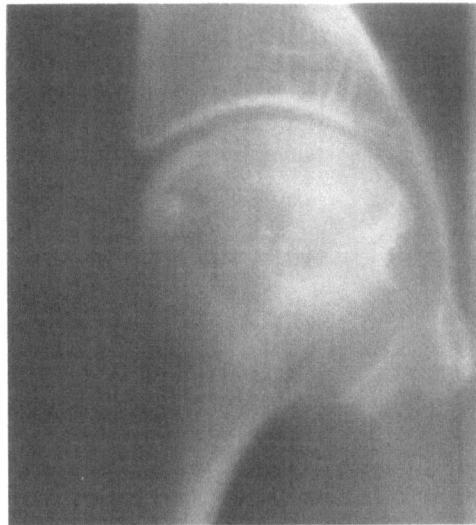

Fig. 10.7. Man aged 32 years with nodular sclerosing HD. One year after initial diagnosis, pelvic films were prompted by vague pain: they showed a mixed, predominantly sclerotic tumor of the left metaphyseal-diaphyseal femur, with destruction and local expansion of the cortical bone. Biopsy revealed a new site of HD

Fig. 10.8. Patient with HD treated by pelvic irradiation and chemotherapy. The patient had pain in the right hip, and CT demonstrated heterogeneous disorganization of the femoral head with slight displacement and the typical appearance of osteonecrosis

ably reflected the fact that bone involvement appeared late in the course of the disease and thus in patients with prolonged survival. Even in the most recent series, hematogenous dissemination carries a somber prognosis.

10.2 Non-Hodgkin's Lymphoma

10.2.1 Mechanism of Appearance

Non-Hodgkin's lymphoma (NHL) causes much more diffuse lesions than HD. While invasion resulting from contiguous extension is possible (Figs. 10.9–10.12), hematogenous dissemination is much more common (Fig. 10.13).

10.2.2 Incidence

Radiologically demonstrable initial lesions occur in around 5% of patients with NHL [295, 597]. Solitary bone lesions constitute a separate entity. Any bone can be affected, but the axial skeleton (the spine, pelvis, ribs, skull, and facial bones) is involved much more often than the extremities.

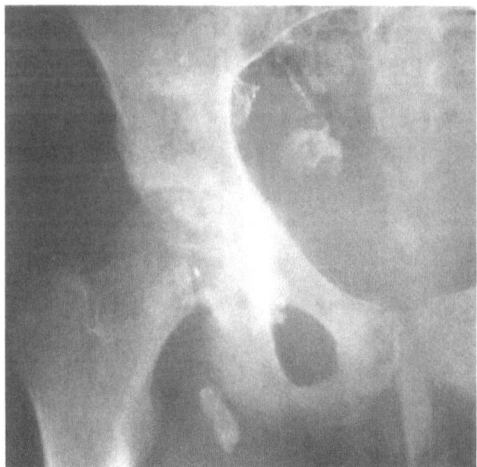

Fig. 10.9. Male patient aged 17 years. Pathological lymphogram revealing right iliac nodes and soft-tissue masses. The right cotyloid cavity is the site of mixed architectural changes resulting from contiguous spread

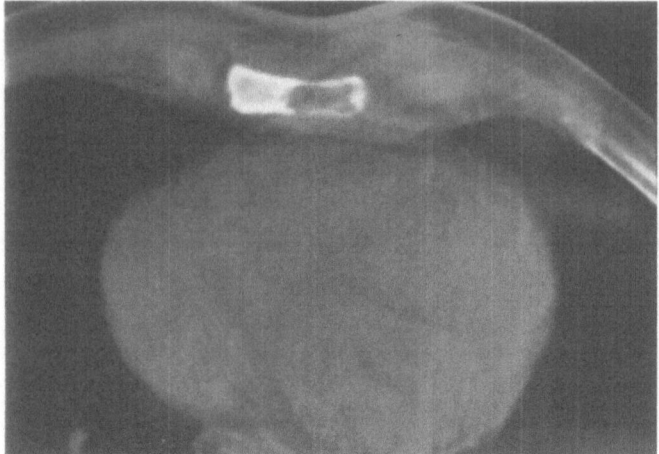

Fig. 10.10. Man aged 28 years with a recently developed presternal mass. Histology study diagnosed NHL. CT demonstrates a left pre- and laterosternal mass causing osteolysis of the left half of the sternum

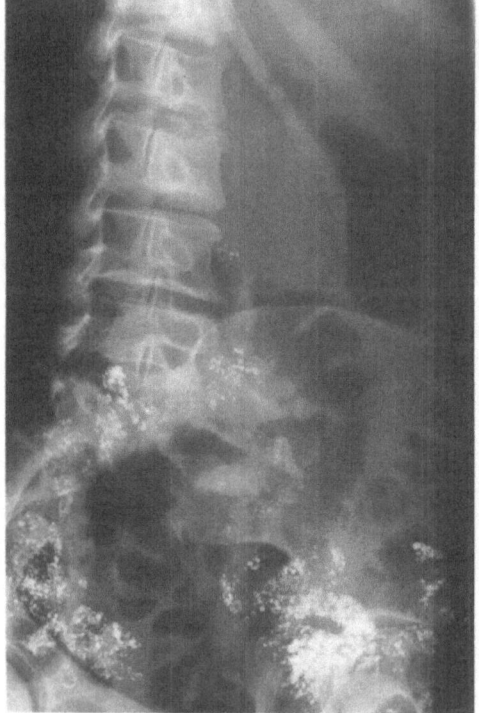

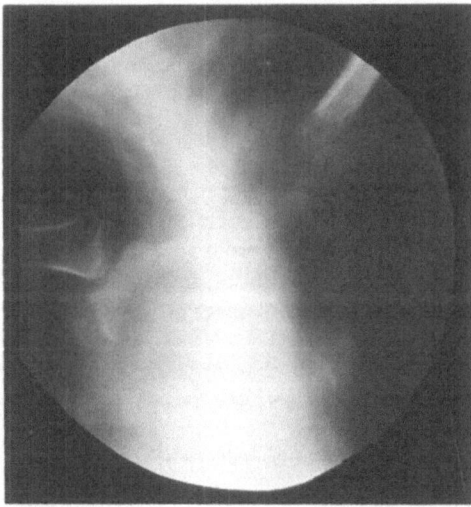

Fig. 10.11. Man aged 48 years with NHL. Lymphography: the irregularly filled opacified nodes are all hypertrophic and clearly pathologic. Osteosclerosis is evident in the bodies of L-1 and L-3

Fig. 10.12. Man aged 39 years with recent appearance of a painful left supraclavicular node. Histology study diagnosed immunoblastic NHL. Frontal tomogram: osteolysis of the body of the sternal manubrium and the medial end of the left clavicle

Involvement is often diffuse, producing the same radiological appearances as in HD (Fig. 10.14). The average age of patients is 40 years. Lesions predominate in the 5th and 6th decades, but can appear at any age.

10.2.3 Radiological Features

While neither complete skeletal surveys nor radionuclide bone scanning are performed on a routine basis, they are indicated for certain histological types [290, 441, 460, 520]. The radiological features vary considerably; lesions are essentially lytic, and bone destruction may be permeative (indicative of very aggressive lesions), moth-eaten, or, less frequently, geographic. The rare instances of periosteal reaction are constituted by discrete thickenings, and en-

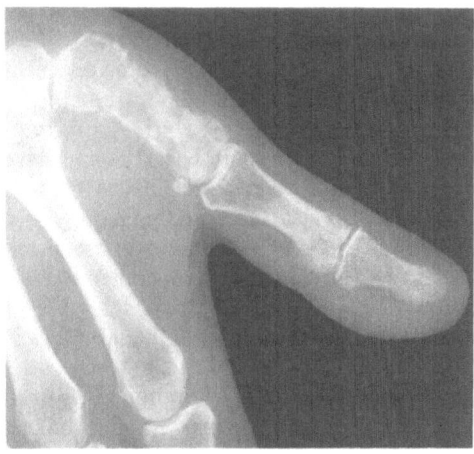

Fig. 10.13. Woman aged 40 years with NHL of the maxillary sinus, presenting with pain in the right thumb. Radiograph shows osteolysis of the first metacarpal; a poorly delimited mixed lesion with cortical destruction and soft-tissue tumor

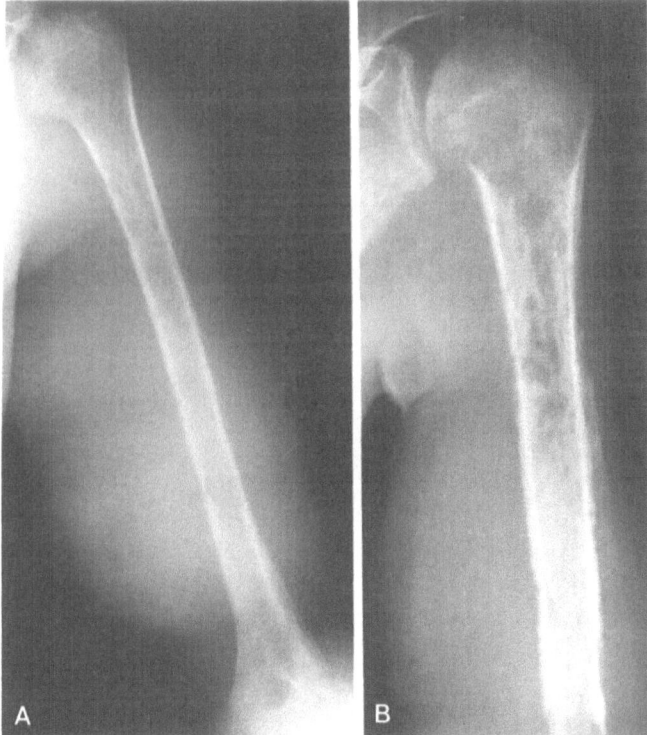

Fig. 10.14 A, B. Man aged 24 years. Pain in the knees, then in the left arm, of 3 months' duration. Recent swelling in left arm, with weight loss and deterioration of general condition. Cutaneous permeation nodules. Histology study revealed diffuse large-cell centroblastic NHL. Bone scan showed the uptake of contrast material in the left humerus and left femur. A The film of the left humerus shows a bulky soft-tissue tumor totally encasing the left humerus, with multiple cortical lesions. B Following chemotherapy, the humeral lesions are much more evident, with cortical destruction and longitudinal periosteal reaction

dosteal thickening can be seen in the cortical bone. The cortical bone can be thinned, but is most often destroyed. Soft-tissue involvement is frequent. Mixed lesions are rare, and purely sclerotic lesions even more so [199]. Fractures are more common than in HD. Attempts have been made to correlate radiological features with the histological type and lesion prognosis. The poorly differentiated and undifferentiated histiocytic lymphomas of Rappaport's classification have been implicated in all types of NHL bone involvement. The other histological types are rarely accompanied by osseous lesions. No correlation has been found between cortical bone destruction and disseminated medullary involvement. Radionuclide bone scanning has proven suitable for initial disease extension work-up. More detailed analysis of lesion features, the cortical bone, periosteal reaction, and soft-tissue involvement has shown the reliability of cortical destruction and soft-tissue invasion in predicting a poor outcome; no prognostic value has been found for cortical thickening or periosteal reaction. Osseous involvement is generally accompanied by medi-

ocre survival (approximately 20% at 5 years) [555, 588, 637]. Solitary diffuse cortical bone lesions, without adenopathies or hepatosplenomegaly, have been reported [128, 629], but remain exceptional (Fig. 10.15).

Primary bone lymphoma (the reticulum cell sarcoma of Parker and Jackson) warrants consideration as a separate entity. There is a marked male predominance (approximately two-thirds of cases). Primary bone lymphoma can occur at any age, but adults are affected most often and lesions are exceptional in children under 10 years of age. The anatomical distribution is also different. Most authors have noted a predilection for the long bones of the extremities [46, 151, 204]: 40% of lesions affect the knee region, the femur, tibia, or humerus. Pelvic, scapular, costal, and vertebral sites are less common (Fig. 10.16).

10.2.4 Clinical Features

Since pain, the most frequent symptom, is often moderate, an interval of several months may

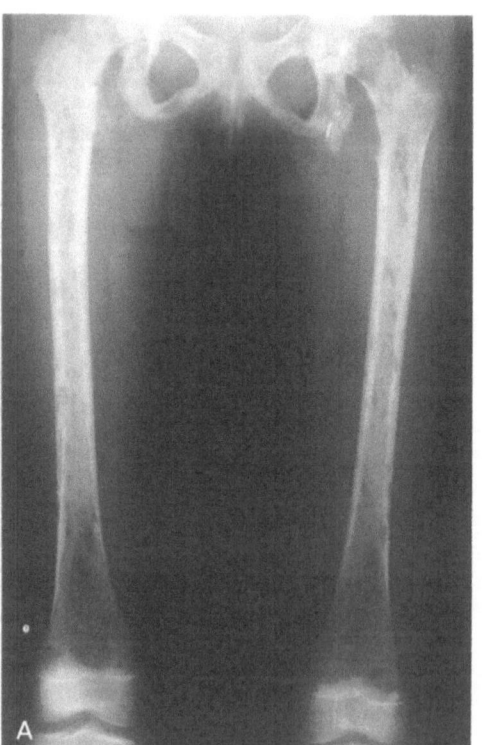

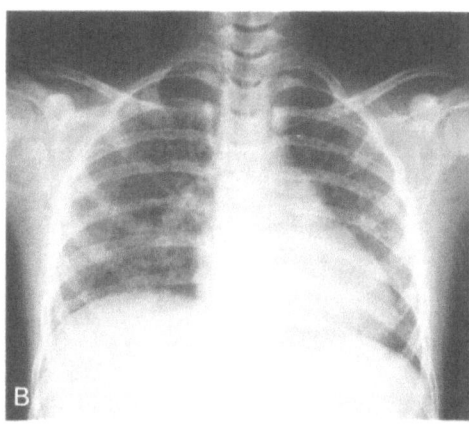

Fig. 10.15 A, B. Girl aged 9 years with diffuse joint pain. Radiological survey [629] revealed multiple well-defined bone lesions centered in the cortical bone, with osteolysis of the right lower trochanter. Bone biopsy disclosed a lymphosarcoma. At the time of discovery, the bone lesions were solitary, without adenopathy or hepatosplenomegaly

elapse before diagnosis. Swelling is rare, whereas distinctive pathological fracture is frequent, since the lesion has been tolerated for an extended period. This disparity between an often bulky lesion and its excellent tolerance is somwhat peculiar to primary bone lymphomas (Fig. 10.17).

Long-bone involvement tends to be metaphyseal rather than diaphyseal, and the lesion is usually lytic. Bone destruction can produce a permeative pattern, but moth-eaten (Fig. 10.18) and geographic patterns are more common. Extension into the cortical bone occurs slowly, often with endosteal thickening and ultimately osteolysis; thick periosteal reactions are frequent. Multiple lamellated reactions, Codman's triangle, and perpendicular periosteal reactions are much rarer. The osteolysis seen in mixed forms is purely reactive and not tumoral (Fig. 10.17). The soft-tissue tumor that ensues once the lesion invades the soft tissues is not ossified. Osseous lymphomas of the knee region can provoke a synovial reaction, which is rare with other tumors. In general, osseous sites of NHL are usually large tumors with a slow growth rate.

Several studies have attempted to correlate radiological features with prognosis [68, 152, 489, 588]. Pathological fracture, periosteal reaction, cortical breakthrough, and soft-tissue tumors

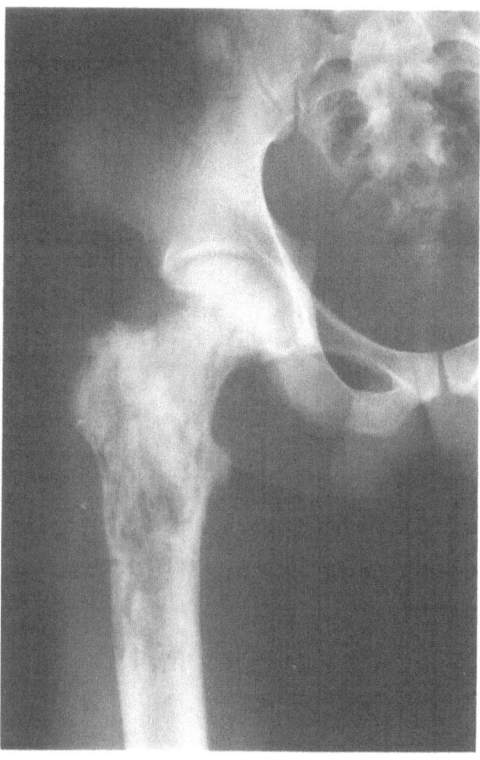

Fig. 10.17. Man aged 30 years with pain of several years' duration. Mixed lytic and sclerotic tumor of the upper third of the femur, from the epiphysis to the diaphysis, with partial destruction of the cortex and rare linear periosteal reactions

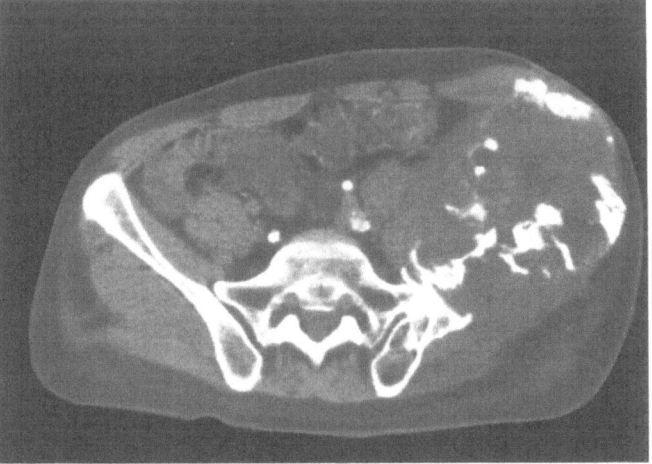

Fig. 10.16. Woman aged 34 years with pain in the left hip. CT scar shows bulky lytic tumor of the left iliac wing, which is almost entirely destroyed, and extensive swelling of the soft-tissue components

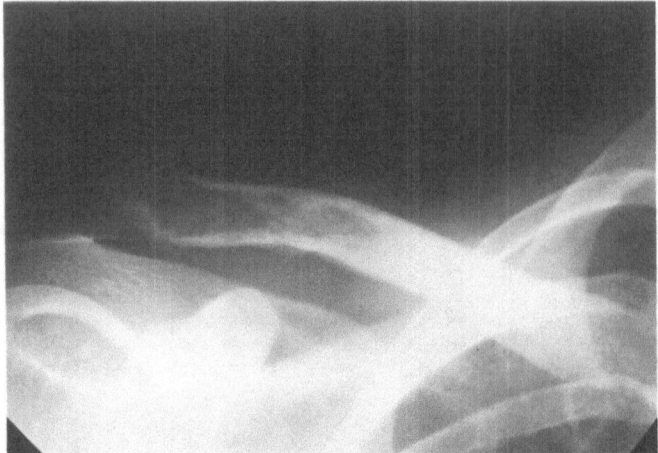

Fig. 10.18. Patient with pain in the outer end of the right clavicle. Film shows pure osteolysis, with moth-eaten destruction of the distal third of the clavicle. Histology study diagnosed NHL

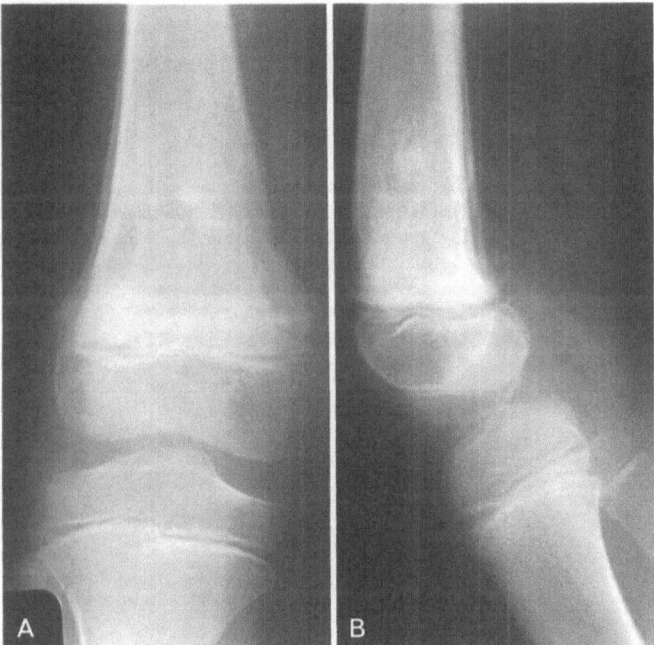

Fig. 10.19 A, B. Boy aged 8 years. Chest radiography showed subcutaneous thoracic nodules and mediastinal adenopathies. The patient had pain in the left knee. Radiographs reveal predominantly sclerotic mixed involvement of the lower metaphyseal femur, with cortical destruction and linear periosteal reaction (note the nonossified fibroma). Node biopsy demonstrated malignant histiocytosis

all seem to be associated with a poor prognosis, whereas the patterns of bone destruction and osteosclerosis appear to be of no predictive value. The differential diagnosis depends on the radiological findings: osteosarcoma, fibrosarcoma, or chondrosarcoma, and especially metastasis or myeloma for lytic forms. Age is a reliable prognostic factor. Staging is the same as for other lymphomas. Primary bone lymphomas are currently considered solitary initial sites of lymphoma. The prognosis is much better than for diffuse lymphomas.

10.3 Burkitt's Lymphoma

Burkitt's lymphoma generally affects children under 10 years of age [98]; the lesions of the facial bones are particularly distinctive.

10.4 Malignant Histiocytosis

Osseous lesions are rare [497, 630]. They can be lytic, with a sclerotic rim, or sclerotic, with the possibility of cortical destruction and periosteal reaction (Fig. 10.19). Lesions of this type can regress with treatment.

11 References

1. Abel WG, Finnerty J (1969) Primary Hodgkin's disease of thyroid. NY State J Med 69: 314-315
2. Abeloff MD, Lenhard RE (1974) Clinical management of ureteral obstruction secondary to malignant lymphoma. Johns Hopkins Med J 134: 34-42
3. Abt AB, Kirschner RH, Belliveau RE, O'Connell MJ, Sklansky BD, Greene WH, Wiernik PH (1974) Hepatic pathology associated with Hodgkin's disease. Cancer 33: 1564-1571
4. Ackerman NB, Aust JC, Bredenberg CE, Hanson VA Jr, Rogers LS (1976) Problems in differentiating between pancreatic lymphoma and anaplastic carcinoma and their management. Ann Surg 184: 705-708
5. Aghai E, Hertz M, Ramot B, Brenner HJ (1978) Hodgkin's disease of the lung. Isr J Med Sci 14: 1019-1025
6. Ahmann DL, Kiely JM, Harrison EG Jr, Payne WS (1966) Malignant lymphoma of the spleen. A review of 49 cases in which the diagnosis was made at splenectomy. Cancer 19: 461-469
7. Aisenberg AC, Long JC (1979) A 54-year old man with nodular lymphoma and circulating atypical lymphocytes. N Engl J Med 301: 1332-1339
8. Alcorn FS, Majegrano VC, Petasnick JP, Clark JW (1977) Contributions of computed tomography in the staging and management of malignant lymphoma. Radiology 125: 717-723
9. Alford BA, Coccia PF, L'Heureux PR (1977) Roentgenographic features of American Burkitt's lymphoma. Radiology 124: 763-770
10. Algers G, Boquist L, Fodstad H, Liliequist B, Singounas E (1981) Hodgkin's disease primarily localized to the brain. Acta Neurochir (Wien) 59: 231-237
11. Al Khateeb AK (1970) Primary malignant lymphoma of the small intestine. Int Surg 54: 295-300
12. Allen Good C (1963) Tumors of the small intestine. Caldwell lecture. Am J Roentgenol 89: 685-705
13. Al Saleem T, Harwick R, Robbins R, Blady JV (1970) Malignant lymphomas of the pharynx. Cancer 26: 1383-1387
14. Ambos MA, Bosniak MA, Madayag MA, Lefleur RS (1977) Infiltrating neoplasms of the kidney. Am J Roentgenol 129: 859-864
15. Anderson HA, Maisel RH, Cantrell RW (1976) Isolated laryngeal lymphoma. Laryngoscope 86: 1251-1257
16. André C, Garel L, Sauvegrain J (1982) Rein et lymphome chez l'enfant: apport de l'échographie. A propos de 9 cas. Ann Radiol 25: 385-394
17. Andrews GA, Hubner KF, Greenlaw RH (1978) Ga-67 citrate imaging in malignant lymphoma: final report of cooperative group. J Nucl Med 19: 1013-1019
18. Andrieu JM, Weh HJ, Teillet F, Jacquillat C, Boiron M (1978) Localisation pulmonaire de la maladie de Hodgkin. Aspects initiaux et évolutions. Nouv Presse Med 7: 3737-3741
19. Applefeld MM, Cole JF, Pollock SH, Sutton FJ, Slawson RG, Singleton RI, Wifrnik AH (1981) The late appearance of chronic pericardial disease in patients treated by radiotherapy for Hodgkin's disease. Ann Intern Med 94: 338-341
20. Aqualina JN, Bugeja TJ (1974) Primary malignant lymphoma of the bladder: case report and review of the literature. J Urol 112: 64-65
21. Arnon S (1975) Lymphographic patterns in lymphoma. West J Med 122: 319-320
22. Aron E, Jobard P, Groussin P, Jankowski JM (1971) Lymphosarcome bilatéral et primitif des glandes surrénales. Sem Hôp Paris 47: 3067-3071
23. Aschner M, Bercu G (1974) Contribution au diagnostic radiologique du lymphosarcome du duodénum. J Radiol 54: 411-412
24. Asher WM, Freimanis AK (1969) Echographic diagnosis of retroperitoneal lymph node enlargement: ultrasonic scanning technique and diagnostic findings. Am J Roentgenol 105: 437-445
25. Balikian JP, Herman PC (1979) Non-Hodgkin lymphoma of the lung. Radiology 132: 569-576
26. Baltaxe H, Watson R, Lerin D (1972) Angiographic appearance of splenic masses. Angiology 23: 316-327
27. Balthazar EJ (1977) The radiology corner. Duodenal Hodgkin's disease. Am J Gastroenterol 68: 306-311
28. Banfi A, Bonadonna G, Carnevali G, Molinari R, Monfardini S, Salvini E (1970) Lymphoreticular sarcomas with primary involvement of Waldeyer's ring. Clinical evaluation of 225 cases. Cancer 26: 341-351

29. Banfi A, Lattuada A, Musumeci R (1974) Lymphography and laparatomy in Hodgkin's disease: their prognostic value and relevance in the therapeutic program. In: Gomez-Lopez J, Bonmanti J (eds) Radiology, Proceedings of the 13th International Congress of Radiology, vol 2. Excerpta Medica, Amsterdam, pp 11-16

30. Banks DE, Castellan RM, Hendrick DJ (1980) Lymphocytic lymphoma recurring in multiple endobronchial sites. Thorax 35: 796-797

31. Barbaric ZL, Mac Intosh PK (1981) Periureteral thin-needle aspiration biopsy. Urol Radiol 2: 181-185

32. Baron RL, Sagel SS, Baglan RJ (1981) Thymic cysts following radiation therapy for Hodgkin's disease. Radiology 141: 593-597

33. Baroni CD, Malchiodi F (1980) Histology, age and sex distribution and pathologic correlations of Hodgkin's disease. A study of 184 cases observed in Rome, Italy. Cancer 45: 1549-1555

34. Baylor SM, Berg JW (1973) Cross-classification and survival characteristics of 5000 cases of cancer of the pancreas. J Surg Oncol 5: 335-358

35. Beachley MC, Lau BP, King ER (1972) Bone involvement in Hodgkin's disease. Am J Roentgenol 114: 559-563

36. Bedikian AY, Khankhanian N, Heilburn LK, Valdivieso M (1980) Primary lymphomas and sarcomas of the stomach. South Med J 73: 21-24

37. Bedivian M, Simu G (1978) Lesions of the female genital tract in leukemia and lymphoma. Morphol Embryol (Bucur) 24: 221-224

38. Belliveau RE, Wiernick PH, Abt AB (1974) Liver enzymes and pathology in Hodgkin's disease. Cancer 34: 300-305

39. Benacerraf R (1974) Apport de l'artériographie digestive au diagnostic des tumeurs du grêle. Ann Radiol 17: 751-764

40. Benfield GFA (1979) Primary lymphosarcoma of lung associated with hypertrophic pulmonary osteoarthropathy. Thorax 34: 279-280

41. Bennett JM (1981) Lymphomas. 1. Including Hodgkin's disease. Nijhoff, The Hague

42. Bennett MH, Farrer-Brown G, Henry K, Jelliffe AM (1974) Classification of non-Hodgkin's lymphomas. Lancet 2: 405-406

43. Beretta G, Spinelli P, Rilke F, Tancini G, Canetta R, Gennari L, Bonadonna G (1976) Sequential laparoscopy and laparotomy combined with bone marrow biopsy in staging Hodgkin's disease. Cancer Treat Rep 60: 1231-1237

44. Bergonzini R, Canossi GC, Ramagnoli R (1968) Localizzazioni emoblastosiche del colon e del retto. Osservazioni radiologische in 18 casi. Nunt Radiol 34: 1215-1239

45. Berman MD, Falchuk KR, Trey C, Gramm HF (1979) Primary histiocytic lymphoma of the esophagus. Dig Dis Sci 24: 883-886

46. Bey P, Stines J, Schoumacher P (1977) Les réticulosarcomes osseux. Les aspects radiologiques à propos de 48 observations. J Radiol 58: 246-247

47. Bisbee AC, Thoeny RH (1975) Malignant lymphoma of the thyroid following irradiation. Cancer 35: 1296-1299

48. Bitran JD, Kinzie J, Sweet DL, Variakojis D, Griem ML, Golomb HM, Miller JB, Oetzel N, Ultmann JE (1977) Survival of patients with localized histiocytic lymphoma. Cancer 39: 342-346

49. Blackledge G, Best JJK, Crowther D, Isherwood I (1980) Computed tomography (CT) in the staging of patients with Hodgkin's disease: a report on 136 patients. Clin Radiol 31: 143-147

50. Blackledge G, Mamtora H, Crowther D, Isherwood I, Best JJ (1981) The role of abdominal computed tomography in lymphoma following treatment. Br J Radiol 54: 955-960

51. Blank N, Castellino RA (1980) Chest. In: Felson B (ed) Roentgenology of the lymphoma and leukemias. Grune and Stratton, New York, pp 30-48

52. Bloch C (1967) Roentgen features of Hodgkin's disease of the stomach. Am J Roentgenol 99: 175-181

53. Boddie AW Jr, Eisemberg BL, Mullins JD, Schlichtemeier AL (1980) The diagnosis and treatment of obstructive jaundice secondary to malignant lymphoma: a problem in multidisciplinary management. J Surg Oncol 14: 111-123

54. Bodin F, Liguory C, Fouet P, Indes J, Conte-Marti J, Conte M (1972) Les infiltrations lymphoïdes primitives. Sem Hôp Paris 48: 167-172

55. Boijsen E, Reuter SR (1966) Mesenteric angiography in the evaluation of inflammatory and neoplastic disease of the intestine. Radiology 87: 1028-1036

56. Boivin JF, Hutchison GB (1982) Coronary heart disease mortality after irradiation for Hodgkin's disease. Cancer 49: 2470-2475

57. Bonnadonna G, Lattuada A, Monfardini S, Milani R, Banfi A (1979) Combined radiotherapy chemotherapy in localized non Hodgkin's lymphoma. Five years results of a randomized study. In: Jones SE, Salmon SE (eds) Adjuvant therapy of cancer. II. Grune and Stratton, New York, pp 145-173

58. Bonzanini C (1974) Linfogranuloma maligno primitivo dello stomaco. Minerva Chir 29: 54-59

59. Bosch EP, Cancilla PA, Cornell SH (1976) CT in progressive multifocal leukoencephalopathy. Arch Neurol 33: 216

60. Bosniak MA, Megibow AJ, Ambos MA, Mitnick JS, Lefleur RS, Gordon R (1982) Computed tomography of ureteral obstruction. Am J Roentgenol 138: 1107-1113

61. Bouroncle BA, Old JW Jr, Vazques AG (1962) Pathogenesis of jaundice in Hodgkin's disease. Arch Int Med 110: 872-883

62. Bouvier M, Lejeune E, Deplante JP, Le Provost C (1975) Les manifestations osseuses révélatrices de la maladie de Hodgkin. Rhumatologie 27: 177-193

63. Brady LW, Asbell SO (1980) Malignant lymphoma of the gastrointestinal tract. Erskine Memorial lecture 1979. Radiology 137: 291-298

64. Brant-Zawadzki M, Enzmann DR (1978) Computed tomographic brain scanning in patients with lymphoma. Radiology 129: 67-71

65. Brasch RC, Royal S, Amman AJ, Crowe J (1979) Pseudolymphoma in two immunodeficient children. Am J Roentgenol 132: 844-847

66. Brascho DJ, Durant JR, Green LE (1977) The accuracy of retroperitoneal ultrasonography in Hodgkin's disease and non-Hodgkin's lymphoma. Radiology 125: 485-487

67. Braunstein EM (1980) Hodgkin disease of bone: radiographic correlation with the histological classification. Radiology 137: 643-646

68. Braunstein EM, White SJ (1980) Non-Hodgkin lymphoma of bone. Radiology 135: 59-63

69. Brazis PW, Biller J, Fine M, Palacios E, Pagano RJ (1981) Cerebellar degeneration with Hodgkin's disease. Arch Neurol 38: 253-256

70. Breiman RS, Castellino RA, Harell GS, Marshall WH, Glatstein E, Kaplan HS (1978) CT-pathologic correlation in Hodgkin's disease and non-Hodgkin's lymphoma. Radiology 126: 159-166

71. Bremen A, Flamand C (1958) Lymphogranulomatose maligne de l'intestin ou maladie de Hodgkin à localisation intestinale primitive. Acta Chir Belg [Suppl]: 99-103

72. Brereton HD, Johnson RE (1974) Calcification in mediastinal lymph nodes after radiation therapy of Hodgkin's disease. Radiology 112: 705-707

73. Briottet J, Boublier L, Rivot G (1966) Lymphosarcome du grêle. J Radiol 11: 663-666

74. Brugère J, Schlienger M, Gérard-Marchant R, Tubiana M, Pouillart P, Cachin Y (1974) Lymphosarcomes et réticulosarcomes des voies aérodigestives supérieures. Histoire naturelle et résultats de la radiothérapie. Bull Cancer 61: 79-92

75. Brunet R, Hoerni B, Trojani M, Marée D, Eghbali H (1981) Les lymphosarcomes digestifs. A propos de 20 cas. Med Chir Dig 10: 25-28

76. Bruneton JN, Le Treut A, De Mascarel HA, Dilhuydy MH, Hoerni B (1979) Lymphography in angio-immunoblastic lymphadenopathy. Br J Radiol 52: 110-115

77. Bruneton JN, Lesbats G, Boublil JL, Fenart D, Aubanel D, Schneider M (1980) Exploration et surveillance du rétropéritoine au cours des lymphomes non hodgkiniens par la lymphographie et l'échographie. J Radiol 61: 779-784

78. Bruneton JN, Caramella E, Boublil JL, Roux P, Abbes M, Demard F (1982) Echographic aspects of thyroid and parotid localizations in non-Hodgkin lymphomas. Fortschr Röntgenstr 136: 530-533

79. Bruneton JN, Thyss A, Bourry J, Bidoli R, Schneider M (1983) Colonic and rectal lymphomas. Report of 6 cases and review of the literature. Fortschr Roentgenstr 138: 283-287

80. Bruneton JN, Roux P, Caramella E, Demard F, Vallicioni J, Chauvel P (1984) Ear, nose and throat cancer. Ultrasound diagnosis of metastasis to cervical lymph nodes. Radiology 152: 771-773

81. Bryan RN, Miller RH, Ferreyro RI, Sessions RB (1982) Computed tomography of the major salivary glands. Am J Roentgenol 139: 547-554

82. Bucy PC, Jerva MJ (1962) Primary epidural spinal lymphosarcoma. J Neurosurg 19: 142-152

83. Bunn PA, Schelchter GP, Jaffe E, Blanay D, Young RL, Mattews MJ, Blattner W, Broder S, Robert-Guroff M, Gallo RC (1983) Clinical course of retrovirus associated adult T-cell lymphoma in the United States. N Engl J Med 309: 257-264

84. Burgener FA, Hamlin DJ (1981) Intrathoracic histiocytic lymphoma. Am J Roentgenol 136: 499-504

85. Burgess JN, Dockerty MB, Remine WH (1971) Sarcomatous lesions of the stomach. Ann Surg 173: 758-766

86. Burke JS, Butler JJ, Fuller LM (1977) Malignant lymphomas of the thyroid. A clinical pathologic study of 35 patients including ultrastructural observations. Cancer 39: 1587-1602

87. Burkitt DP, O'Connor GT (1961) Malignant lymphoma in African children. I. A clinical syndrome. Cancer 14: 258-269

88. Bush RS, Ash CL (1969) Primary lymphoma of the gastrointestinal tract. Radiology 92: 1349-1354

89. Buy JN, Moss AA (1982) Computed tomography of gastric lymphoma. Am J Roentgenol 138: 859-865

90. Byrne GE (1977) Rappaport classification of non Hodgkin's lymphoma: histologic features and clinical significance. Cancer Treat Rep 61: 935-944

91. Cabanillas F, Zornoza J, Haynie TP, Rodriguez V (1977) Comparison of lymphangiograms and gallium scans in the non-Hodgkin's lymphomas. Cancer 39: 85-88

92. Cabanillas FL, Bodey GP, Freireich EJ (1980) Management with chemotherapy only of stage I and II malignant lymphoma of aggressive histologic types. Cancer 46: 2356-2359

93. Cachin Y, Brugère J, Gérard-Marchant R, Pierquin B, Richard J (1966) Lymphosarcomes et réticulosarcomes de la région cervico-faciale. A propos 107 cas de formes apparemment localisées, traités et suivis à l'Institut Gustave Roussy, 1951-1964. Sem Hôp Paris 42: 3173-3182

94. Cachin Y, Brugère J, Schaab G (1978) Les localisations cervico-faciales (ORL et buccales) des lymphomes malins non-Hodgkiniens. Vie Med 17: 1551-1560

95. Cadotte M, Brochu P, Verdy M (1971) La glande thyroïde. III. Revue de 100 cas de cancer. Union Med Can 100: 267-270

96. Calenoff L (1972) Gastrointestinal Kaposi's sarcoma: roentgen manifestations. Am J Roentgenol 114: 525-528

97. Camino FA, Colunga F (1974) Linfoma del cervix uterino (informe de dos casos). Ginecol Obstet Mex 36: 41-47

98. Canady JH, Arremds NW (1964) Analysis of 965 tumors seen in patients below age 15. JAMA 64: 59

99. Capron JP, Marti R, Delamarre J (1976) Réticulosarcome jéjunal compliquant une maladie coeliaque de l'adulte. Nouv Presse Med 5: 80-82

100. Carbone PP, Kaplan HS, Musshoff K, Smithers DW, Tubiana M (1971) Report of the Committee on Hodgkin's disease staging classification. Cancer Res 31: 1860-1861

101. Carnovale RL, Goldstein HM, Zornoza J, Dodd GD (1977) Radiologic manifestations of esophageal lymphoma. Am J Roentgenol 128: 751-754

102. Carnovale RL, Zornoza J, Goldman AM, Luna M (1977) Pulmonary alveolar proteinosis: its association with hematologic malignancies and lymphoma. Radiology 122: 303-306

103. Caron J, Delahaye RP, Caron-Poitreau C (1977) Les affections ganglionnaires du médiastin. In: Bismuth V, Bléry M, Rémy J, Caron J, Coulomb M (eds) Traité de radiodiagnostic, Vol IV-1. Masson, Paris, pp 390-395

104. Carroll BA (1981) Lymphoma. In: Goldberg BB (ed) Ultrasound in cancer. Churchill Livingstone, New York, pp 52-67

105. Carroll BA, Lane B, Norman D, Enzmann D (1977) Diagnosis of progressive multifocal leukoencephalopathy by CT. Radiology 122: 137-141

106. Carroll BA, Han NTA (1980) The ultrasonic appearance of extranodal abdominal lymphoma. Radiology 136: 419-425

107. Caruso, RD, Berk RN (1970) Lymphoma of the esophagus. Radiology 95: 381-382

108. Cassady JR, Sagerman RH, Chang CH (1967) Radiation therapy for lymphoma of the spinal canal. Radiology 89: 313-315

109. Castaldo TW, Ballon SC, Lagasse LD, Petrilli ES (1979) Reticuloendothelial neoplasia of the female genital tract. Obstet Gynecol 54: 167-170

110. Castaneda-Zuniga WR, Amplatz K (1977) Angiography of the liver in lymphoma. Radiology 122: 679-681

111. Castellino RA (1974) Observations on "reactive (follicular) hyperplasia" as encountered in repeat lymphography in the lymphomas. Cancer 34: 2042-2050

112. Castellino RA, Blank N, Cassady JR, Kaplan HS (1973) Roentgenologic aspects of Hodgkin's disease. II. Role of routine radiographs in detecting initial relapse. Cancer 31: 316-323

113. Castellino RA, Fuks Z, Blank N, Kaplan HS (1973) Roentgenologic aspects of Hodgkin's disease: repeat lymphangiography. Radiology 109: 53-58

114. Castellino RA, Billingham M, Dorfman RF (1974) Lymphographic accuracy in Hodgkin's disease and malignant lymphoma with a note on the "reactive" lymph node as a cause of most false-positive lymphograms. Invest Radiol 9: 155-165

115. Castellino RA, Glastein E, Turbow MM, Rosenberg S, Kaplan HS (1974) Latent radiation injury of lungs or heart activated by steroid withdrawal. Ann Intern Med 80: 593-599

116. Castellino RA, Goffinet DR, Blank N, Parker BR, Kaplan HS (1974) The role of radiography in the staging of non-Hodgkin's lymphoma with laparotomy correlation. Radiology 110: 329-338

117. Castellino RA, Fossati Bellami F, Gasparini M, Musumeci R (1975) Radiologic findings in previously untreated children with non-Hodgkin's lymphoma. Radiology 117: 657-663

118. Castellino RA, Filly R, Blanck N (1976) Routine full-lung tomography in the initial staging and treatment planning of patients with Hodgkin's disease and non-Hodgkin's lymphoma. Cancer 38: 1130-1136

119. Castellino RA, Marglin SI, Blank N (1980) Retroperitoneum. In: Felson B (ed) Roentgenology of the lymphomas and leukemias. Grune and Stratton, London, pp 80-93

120. Castellino RA, Marglin SI, Carroll BA, Young SW, Harell GS, Blank N (1980) The radiographic evaluation of abdominal and pelvic lymph nodes in oncologic practice. Cancer Treat Rev 7: 153-160

121. Castellino RA, Hoppe RT, Blank N, Young SW, Neumann C, Rosenberg SA, Kaplan HS (1984) Computed tomography, lymphography, and staging laparotomy: correlations in initial staging of Hodgkin disease. Am J Roentgenol 143: 37-41

122. Chabloz R, Givel JL, Saraga P, Saegesser F (1980) Lymphomes et pseudo-lymphomes gastriques. Helv Chir Acta 47: 547-553

123. Chabner BA, Johnson RE, Young RL (1976) Segmental nonsurgical and surgical staging of non Hodgkin's lymphoma. Ann Inter Med 85: 149-154

124. Chadli A, Lennert K (1979) Les lymphomes malins non-hodgkiniens du tube digestif. Ann Anat Pathol (Paris) 24: 231-250

125. Chak LY, Hoppe RT, Burke JS, Kaplan HS (1981) Non-Hodgkin's lymphoma presenting as thyroid enlargement. Cancer 48: 2712-2716

126. Chan KW, Miller DR, Rosen G, Tan CTC (1982) Hodgkin's disease in adolescents presenting as a primary bone lesion. A report of four cases and review of literature. Am J Pediatr Hematol Oncol 4: 11–17

127. Chilcote WA, Borkowski GP (1983) Computed tomography in renal lymphoma. J Comput Assist Tomogr 7: 439–443

128. Child JA, Smith IE (1975) Lymphoma presenting as "idiopathic juvenile osteoporosis". Br Med J 1: 720–721

129. Chorlton I, Norris HJ, King FM (1974) Malignant reticuloendothelial disease involving the ovary as a primary manifestation. A series of 19 lymphomas and 1 granulocytic sarcoma. Cancer 34: 397–407

130. Chou ST, Arkles LB, Gill GB, Pinkus N, Parkin A, Hicks JD (1983) Primary lymphoma of the heart. A case report. Cancer 52: 744–747

131. Chuang VP, Bree RL, Bookstein JJ (1974) Angiographic features of focal lymphoma of the liver. Radiology 111: 53–55

132. Clark AW, Cohen SR, Nissenblatt MJ, Wilson SK (1982) Paraplegia following intrathecal chemotherapy. Neuropathologic findings and elevation of myelin basic protein. Cancer 50: 42–47

133. Coggon DNM, Rose DA, Ansell ID (1981) A large bowel lymphoma complicating renal transplantation. Br J Radiol 54: 418–420

134. Cohen N, Canter JW (1959) Hodgkin's disease of the small intestine. Report of six cases. Am J Dig Dis 4: 361–376

135. Cohen WM, Freed SZ, Hasson J (1974) Metastatic cancer to the ureter: a review of the literature and case presentations. J Urol 112: 188

136. Cole P, Mac Mahon B, Aisenberg A (1968) Mortality from Hodgkin's disease in the United States: evidence for the multiple aetiology hypothesis. Lancet 2: 1371–1376

137. Coleman M, Lightdale CJ, Vinciguerra VP, Degnan TJ, Goldstein M, Horwitz ST, Winawer SJ, Silver RT (1976) Peritoneoscopy in Hodgkin disease: confirmations of results by laparotomy. JAMA 236: 2634–2636

138. Collins SM, Hamilton JD, Lewis TD, Laufer I (1978) Small-bowel malabsorption and gastrointestinal malignancy. Radiology 126: 603–609

139. Connors J, Wise L (1974) Management of gastric lymphomas. Am J Surg 127: 102–108

140. Conomy JP, Weinstein MA, Agamanolis D, Holt WS (1976) Computed tomography in progressive multifocal leukoencephalopathy. Am J Roentgenol 127: 663–665

141. Contreary K, Nance FC, Becker WF (1980) Primary lymphoma of the gastrointestinal tract. Ann Surg 191: 593–598

142. Cornes JS (1961) Multiple lymphomatous polyposis of the gastrointestinal tract. Cancer 14: 249–257

143. Costello P, Mauch P (1979) Radiographic features of recurrent intrathoracic Hodgkin's disease following radiation therapy. Am J Roentgenol 133: 201–206

144. Cotman HE, Bloomfield CD, Amplatz K, Sosin H, Kvisk H, Levitt SH (1978) Lymphography as a guide during laparotomy in Hodgkin's and non-Hodgkin's lymphomas. Acta Radiol [Ther] 17: 296–304

145. Craig O, Gregson R (1981) Primary lymphoma of the gastrointestinal tract. Clin Radiol 32: 63–71

146. Crismer R, Lefebvre F, Naome J, Herion F, Delforge M (1970) Maladie de Hodgkin primitive de l'intestin grêle se présentant sous la forme de sténoses étagées du duodénum, du jéjunum et de l'iléon. Sem Hôp Paris 46: 1226–1228

147. Crisp WE, Surwit EA, Grogan TM, Freedam MF (1982) Malignant pelvic lymphoma. Am J Obstet Gynecol 143: 69–74

148. Croizat P, Papillon J, Revol L, Chassard JL, Quinard J (1962) Deux cas de localisation oesophagienne de la lymphogranulomatose maligne. J Radiol 43: 223–227

149. Crowther D, Blackledge G, Best JK (1979) The role of computed tomography of the abdomen in the staging of patients with lymphoma. Clin Haematol 8: 567–591

150. Cupps RE, Hodgson JR, Dockerty MB, Adson MA (1969) Primary lymphoma in the small intestine: problems of roentgenologic diagnosis. Radiology 92: 1355–1362

151. Dahlin DC (1978) Bone tumors: general aspects and data on 6221 cases, 3rd edn. Thomas, Springfield

152. Dalinka MK (1983) Primary lymphoma of bone: radiographic appearance and prognosis. Radiology 147: 288

153. Davey FR, Skarin AT, Moloney WC (1973) Pathology of splenic lymphoma. Am J Clin Pathol 59: 95–103

154. Dawson IMP, Cornes JS, Morson BC (1961) Primary malignant lymphoid tumours of the intestinal tract. Report of 37 cases with a study of factors influencing prognosis. Br J Surg 49: 80–89

155. Debray C, Leymarios J, Comandi A, Benvestito V (1970) La lymphosarcomatose digestive diffuse. A propos de 6 observations. Arch Fr Mal App Dig 59: 178–179

156. De Cosse JJ, Berg JW, Fracchia AA, Farrow JH (1962) Primary lymphosarcoma of the breast: a review of 14 cases. Cancer 15: 1264–1268

157. Deeble TJ, Goldberg DM (1980) Assessment of biochemical tests for bone and liver involvement in malignant lymphoma patients. Cancer 45: 1451–1457

158. De Giuli E, De Giuli G (1977) Lymph node calcification in Hodgkin's disease following irradiation. Acta Radiol [Diagn] 16: 305–313

159. Delahaye RP, Isnard J, Pyard M (1963) Les lymphosarcomes du caecum. J Radiol 44: 625–634

160. Delumeau G, Toscer L (1971) Localisation gastrique de la maladie de Hodgkin. Sem Hôp Paris 47: 1496-1498

161. De Santo LW, Weiland LH (1970) Malignant lymphoma of the larynx. Laryngoscope 80: 966-978

162. De Smet AA, Tubergen DG, Martel W (1976) Nodular lymphoid hyperplasia of the colon associated with dysgammaglobulinemia. Am J Roentgenol 127: 515-517

163. Devers L (1979) Valeur-pronostique des localisations osseuses initales dans la maladie de Hodgkin. A propos de 17 cas. Thesis, Paris

164. De Vita VT Jr (1982) Hodgkin's disease: conference summary and future directions. Cancer Treat Rep 66: 1045-1055

165. Dhermy P (1978) Considération sur les classifications actuelles des tumeurs lymphoïdes orbito-palpébrales. Bulletin de la Société ophtalmologique de Paris 2: 847-850

166. Dickson R (1971) Lymphoma of the larynx. Laryngoscope 81: 578-585

167. Diebold J (1974) Classification morphologique des hématosarcomes lymphoïdes non hodgkiniens. Nouv Presse Med 3: 1818

168. Doll DC, Weiss RB, Shah S (1978) Lymphoma of the prostate presenting as benign prostatic hypertrophy. South Med J 71: 1170-1171

169. Dorfman RF (1974) Classification of non Hodgkin's lymphomas. Lancet 1: 1295-1296

170. Dubois PJ, Martinez AJ, Myerowitz RL, Rosenbaum AE (1978) Subependymal and leptomeningeal spread of systemic malignant lymphoma demonstrated by cranial CT. J Comput Assist Tomogr 2: 218-228

171. Dumbadze I, Crawford ED, Mulvaney WP (1979) Lymphomatoid tumor infiltration of renal veins. J Urol 121: 88-89

172. Duncan PR, Checa F, Gowing NF, Mac Elwain TJ, Peckham MJ (1980) Extranodal non Hodgkin's lymphoma presenting in the testicle. A clinical and pathologic study of 24 cases. Cancer 45: 1578-1584

173. Dunnick NR, Fuks Z, Castellino RA (1975) Repeat lymphography in non-Hodgkin's lymphoma. Radiology 115: 349-354

174. Dunnick NR, Parker BR, Castellino RA (1976) Rapid onset of pulmonary infiltration due to histiocytic lymphoma. Radiology 118: 281-285

175. Dunnick NR, Parker BR, Warnke RA, Castellino RA (1976) Radiographic manifestations of malignant histiocytosis. Am J Roentgenol 127: 611-616

176. Dunnick NR, Reaman GH, Head GL, Shawker TH, Ziegler JL (1979) Radiographic manifestations of Burkitt's lymphoma in American patients. Am J Roentgenol 132: 1-6

177. Durkin W, Durant J (1979) Benign mass lesions after therapy for Hodgkin's disease. Arch Intern Med 139: 333-336

178. Edwards RT (1969) Hodgkin's sarcoma of the small bowel. Virginia Medical Monthly 96: 521-525

179. Efsinkd L, Wexels P (1952) Hodgkin's disease of the lung with cavitation. Report of three cases. J Thor Surg 23: 377-387

180. Egeli RA, Quan SH (1980) Lymphome malin primaire du gros intestin. Schweiz Med Wochenschr 110: 1045-1047

181. Ehrlich AN, Stalder G, Geller W, Sherlock P (1968) Gastrointestinal manifestations of malignant lymphoma. Gastroenterology 54: 1115-1121

182. Elie G, Rabin A, Drouillard J, Bruneton JN, Delorme G (1978) Artériographie des tumeurs malignes primitives de la rate. Intérêt, limites. Ann Radiol 21: 591-596

183. Ellert J, Kreel L (1980) The role of computed tomography in the initial staging and subsequent management of the lymphomas. J Comput Assist Tomogr 4: 368-391

184. Engel IA, Straus DJ, Lacher M, Lane J, Smith J (1981) Osteonecrosis in patients with malignant lymphoma: a review of twenty-five cases. Cancer 48: 1243-1250

185. Ennuyer A, Bataini YP (1966) Lymphoréticulosarcomes de l'estomac et de l'intestin. J Radiol 47: 163-175

186. Ennuyer A, Bataini YP (1966) Les tumeurs de l'amygdale et de la région vélopalatine. Masson, Paris

187. Ennuyer A, Bataini P, Helary J (1961) Maladie de Hodgkin des voies aérodigestives supérieures. Ann Oto-Laryng Paris 78: 474-482

188. Enzmann DR, Krikorian J, Norman D, Kramer R, Pollock J, Faer M (1979) CT in primary reticulum cell sarcoma of the brain. Radiology 130: 165-170

189. Enzmann DR, Brant-Zawadzki M, Britt RH (1980) CT of central nervous system infections in immunocompromised patients. Am J Roentgenol 135: 263-267

190. Escudero-Barrilero A, Borruel JLS, Martinez-Pineiro JA (1974) Lymphome rénal. Valeur de l'artériographie sélective. J Urol Nephrol 5: 501-509

191. Evans HL, Butler JJ, Younèss EL (1978) Malignant lymphoma, small lymphocytic type. A clinicopathologic study of 84 cases with suggested criteria for intermediate lymphocytic lymphoma. Cancer 41: 1440-1455

192. Fabian CE, Nudelman EJ, Abrams HL (1966) Postlymphangiogram film as an indicator of tumor activity in lymphoma. Invest Radiol 1: 386-393

193. Faer MJ, Mead JH, Lynch RD (1977) Cerebral granulomatous angiitis: case report and literature review. Am J Roentgenol 129: 463-467

194. Fajardo LF, Eltringham JR, Stewart JR (1976) Combined cardiotoxicity of adriamycin and X-radiation. Lab Invest 34: 84-96

195. Fayos JV, Lampe IA (1971) Cardiac apical mass in Hodgkin's disease. Radiology 99: 15-18

196. Federman J, Goldstein ME, Weingarten (1963) Malignant lymphoma of over 15 years' duration masquerading as ulcerative colitis. Am J Roentgenol 89: 771-778

197. Feld R, Bodey GP (1977) Infections in patients with malignant lymphoma treated with combination chemotherapy. Cancer 39: 1018-1025

198. Felson B (1973) Chest roentgenology. Saunders, Philadelphia

199. Ferrant A, Rodhain J, Michaux JL, Piret L, Maldague B, Sokal G (1975) Detection of skeletal involvement in Hodgkin's disease. A comparison of radiography, bone scanning, and bone marrow biopsy in 38 patients. Cancer 35: 1346-1353

200. Fierstein JT, Thawley SE (1978) Lymphoma of the head and neck. Laryngoscope 88: 582-593

201. Filly R, Blank N, Castellino RA (1976) Radiographic distribution of intrathoracic disease in previously untreated patients with Hodgkin's lymphoma disease and non-Hodgkin's lymphoma. Radiology 120: 277-281

202. Filly RA, Marglin S, Castellino RA (1976) The ultrasonographic spectrum of abdominal and pelvic Hodgkin's disease and non-Hodgkin's disease. Cancer 38: 2143-2148

203. Fiz G, Vital C (1971) A propos d'une localisation gastrique au cours de la maladie de Hodgkin. Bordeaux Med 2: 399-404

204. Foley WD, Baum KJ, Wheeler RH (1975) Diffuse osteosclerosis with lymphocytic lymphoma. A case report. Radiology 117: 553-554

205. Fontaine R, Warter P, Weill F (1961) Aspect radiologique des sarcomes de l'estomac (à propos de 12 observations). J Radiol 42: 509-517

206. Foon KA, Schroff RW, Gale RP (1982) Surface markers on leukemia and lymphoma cells: recent advances. Blood 60: 1-13

207. Forbes WSC, Isherwood I, Fawcitt RA (1978) Computed tomography in the evaluation of the solitary or unilateral nonfunctioning kidney. J Comput Assist Tomogr 2: 389-394

208. Foucar K, Armitage JO, Dick FR (1983) Malignant lymphoma, diffuse mixed small and large cell. A clinicopathologic study of 47 cases. Cancer 51: 2090-2099

209. Franchini A, Tonielli E, Calo G (1979) Le localizzazioni gastrointestinali dei linfomi maligni. Minerva Chir 34: 457-466

210. Frazell EL, Lucas YC (1962) Cancer of the tongue (report of the management of 1554 patients). Cancer 15: 1085-1099

211. Frazer JW Jr (1959) Malignant lymphomas of the gastrointestinal tract. Surg Gynecol Obstet 108: 182-190

212. Freeman C, Berg JW, Cutler SJ (1972) Occurence and prognosis of extranodal lymphomas. Cancer 29: 252-260

213. Friedman M, Kim TH, Panahon AM (1976) Spinal cord compression in malignant lymphoma. Cancer 37: 1485-1491

214. Friedmann AI (1959) Primary lymphosarcoma of the stomach. A clinical study of seventy-five cases. Am J Med 26: 783-896

215. Fu YS, Perkin KH (1972) Lymphosarcoma of the small intestine. A clinicopathologic study. Cancer 29: 645-659

216. Fu YS, Perkin KH (1979) Nonepithelial tumors of the nasal cavity, paranasal sinuses and nasopharynx. A clinicopathologic study. X. Malignant lymphomas. Cancer 43: 611-621

217. Fujii K, Yamagata S, Suzuki J, Sasaki R, Shoji T, Makabe M, Memezawa H, Maesawa H (1972) Angiographic features of submucosal tumors of the stomach. Tohoku J Exp Med 107: 287-299

218. Fuller LM, Gamble JF, Ibrahim E, Jing BS, Butler JJ, Shullemberger CC (1973) Stage II Hodgkin's disease. Significance of mediastinal and nonmediastinal presentations. Radiology 109: 429-435

219. Furnemont E (1976) Localisation gastrique de la lymphoréticulose maligne. A propos d'une observation. Acta Gastroenterol Belg 39: 251-260

220. Gardeur D (1983) Tomodensitométrie intracrânienne. Volume I. Pathologies infectieuses. Ellipses, Paris

221. Gardeur D (1983) Tomodensitométrie craniocérébrale. Volume III. Pathologies neurologiques. Ellipses, Paris

222. Garrett MJ (1981) Complications in the management of the malignant lymphomas (report no. 15). Clin Radiol 32: 537-542

223. Garvie NW, Chu JMG, Nuttall J, Mac Cready VR (1978) Renal involvement with non-Hodgkin's lymphoma: investigation of a recent case. Br J Radiol 51: 547-548

224. Gastaut JA, Gastaut JL, Carcassonne Y (1978) Computerized axial tomography in the study of intracranial complication in hematology. Cancer 41: 487-501

225. Gates GA (1972) Radiosialographic aspects of salivary gland disorders. Laryngoscope 82: 115-130

226. Gaucher P, Floquet J, Bigard MA, Puchelle JC, Fourati R (1972) Localisation hodgkinienne jéjunale isolée. Tunis Med 50: 57-59

227. Gauthier-Benoit C, Houcke M, Demonchy R (1977) Localisation à l'intestin grêle de la maladie de Hodgkin. Lille Med 22: 774-777

228. Gebauer C (1982) Primary lymphosarcoma of the lungs. A review of 121 cases. Oncology 39: 345-349

229. Geboes K, Bossaert H, Dooms MT, Helewaut J (1980) Primary Hodgkin's disease of the stomach in a 72 year old man. J Am Geriatr Soc 28: 71-75

230. Gerard-Marchant R, Hamlin I, Lennert K, Rilke F, Stansfeld AG, Van Unnik JAM (1974) Classi-

fication of non-Hodgkin's lymphomas. Lancet 2: 406–408

231. Gibson JM, Prinn MG (1968) Hodgkin's disease involving the thyroid gland. Br J Surg 55: 236–238

232. Ginaldi S, Bernardino ME, Jing BS, Green B (1980) Ultrasonographic patterns of hepatic lymphoma. Radiology 136: 427–431

233. Givler RL, Brunk SF, Hass CA, Gulesserian HP (1971) Problems of interpretation of liver biopsy in Hodgkin's disease. Cancer 28: 1335–1342

234. Glatstein E, Guernsey JM, Rosenberg SA, Kaplan HS (1969) The value of laparotomy and splenectomy in the staging of Hodgkin's disease. Cancer 24: 709–718

235. Glees JP, Gazet JC, Mac Donald JS, Peckham MJ (1974) The accuracy of lymphography in Hodgkin's disease. Clin Radiol 25: 5–11

236. Goffinet DR, Castellino RA, Kim H, Dorfman RF, Fuks Z, Rosenberg SA, Nelsen T, Kaplan HS (1973) Staging laparotomies in unselected previously untreated patients with non-Hodgkin's lymphomas. Cancer 32: 672–681

237. Goffinet DR, Warnke R, Dunnick NR, Castellino R, Glatstein EJ, Nelson TS, Dorfman RF, Rosenberg SA, Kaplan HS (1977) Clinical and surgical (laparotomy) evaluation of patients with non-Hodgkin's lymphomas. Cancer Treat Rep 61: 981–992

238. Golding S (1982) Computed tomography in the diagnosis of parotid gland tumours. Br J Radiol 55: 182–188

239. Golub GR, Lefemine AA (1969) Multiple malignancies in lymphoproliferative disorders diagnosed by needle aspiration biopsy of pulmonary lesions. Cancer 23: 725–729

240. Goswami AP (1977) Metastatic cancer to the ureter and kidney from malignant lymphoma. A review of the literature. J Urol 117: 381–382

241. Gothlin JH (1976) Post-lymphographic percutaneous fine needle biopsy of lymph nodes guided by fluoroscopy. Radiology 120: 205–207

242. Goudemand M, Wallaert C, Spy E, Sautiere-Habay D (1966) Atteinte caecale au cours d'un lymphosarcome. Lille Med 11: 1001–1005

243. Gowing NFC (1973) Modes of death and post mortem studies. In: Smithers D (ed) Hodgkin's disease. Churchill Livingstone, Edinburgh, pp 163–166

244. Granger W, Whitaker R (1967) Hodgkin's disease in bone with special reference to periostal reaction. Br J Radiol 40: 939–948

245. Grebbel FS, Lyons AR (1971) A further case of lymph node calcification in Hodgkin's disease following radiotherapy. Br J Radiol 44: 720–723

246. Greco AF, Kolins J, Rajjoub RK, Brereton HD (1976) Hodgkin's disease and granulomatous angiitis of the central nervous system. Cancer 38: 2027–2032

247. Green B, Libshitz HI (1979) Bladder and ureter.

In: Libshitz HI (ed) Diagnostic radiology of radiotherapy change. Williams and Wilkins, Baltimore, pp 123–136

248. Green JA, Dawson AA, Jones PF, Brunt PW (1979) The presentation of gastrointestinal lymphoma: study of a population. Br J Surg 66: 798–801

249. Gregory A, Behan M (1981) Lymphoma of the kidneys: unusual ultrasound appearance due to infiltration of the renal sinus. J Clin Ultrasound 9: 343–345

250. Gregory JJ, Ribaudo CA, Grace WJ (1965) Endobronchial Hodgkin's disease. Ann Intern Med 62: 579–586

251. Gros CM, Marion C (1972) Les lymphomes malins du sein. J Belge Radiol 55: 79–86

252. Grossmann H, Winchester PH, Bragg DG, Tan C, Murphy ML (1970) Roentgenographic changes in childhood Hodgkin's disease. Am J Roentgenol 108: 354–364

253. Guardia J, Pedreira JD, Villagrasa M, Allende H, Armengol-Miro JR (1979) Linfomas y seudolinfomas gastricos. Estudio clinico. Med Clin (Barcelona) 72: 54–56

254. Guest JL Jr (1961) Lymphosarcoma of the stomach: a review and analysis of 21 cases. South Med J 54: 175–179

255. Gutman RF, Saavedra JA (1968) Primary Hodgkin's disease of the lung. Report of a case. Dis Chest 34: 660

256. Habib MA, Donaldson JC, Burningham RA (1973) Hodgkin's disease of the colon. South Med J 66: 1067–1068

257. Haddad P, Thaell JF, Kielly JM, Harrison EG Jr, Miller RH (1976) Lymphoma of the spinal extradural space. Cancer 38: 1862–1866

258. Hahn FJY, Peterson N (1977) Renal lymphoma simulating adult polycystic disease. Radiology 122: 655–656

259. Hampel N, Richter-Levin D, Gersh I (1977) Primary lymphosarcoma of prostate. Urology 9: 461–463

260. Harell GS, Breiman RS, Glatstein EJ, Marhall WH Jr, Castellino RA (1977) Computed tomography of the abdomen in the malignant lymphomas. Radiol Clin North Am 15: 391–400

261. Harned RK, Sorrell MF (1978) Hodgkin's disease of the rectum. Radiology 120: 319–320

262. Harnsberger HR, Armstrong JD (1983) Bilateral superomedial hilar displacement: a unique sign of previous mediastinal radiation. Radiology 147: 35–36

263. Harousseau JL, Tricot G, Gisselbrecht C, Asselain B, Flandrin G (1982) Les lymphomes médiastinaux de l'adulte. Etude clinique et histologique de 30 cas. Nouv Presse Med 11: 1393–1396

264. Harousseau JL, Vallantin X, Tricot G, Gisselbrecht C, Jacquillat C (1983) Les localisations neuro-méningées au cours des lymphomes non-

hodgkiniens de l'adulte. Sem Hôp Paris 59: 221–225

265. Harper PG, Fisher C, Mc Lennan K, Souhami RL (1984) Presentation of Hodgkin's disease as an endobronchial lesion. Cancer 53: 147–150

266. Harris ARC, Herrmann RP, Carroll J (1976) Extensive primary lymphoma of the gastrointestinal tract. Aust NZJ Med 6: 571–575

267. Hartman DS, Davis CJ, Goldman SM, Friedman AC, Fritzche P (1982) Renal lymphoma: radiologic-pathologic correlation of 21 cases. Radiology 144: 759–766

268. Haughton VM, Williams AL (1982) Computed tomography of the spine. Mosby, St Louis

269. Haye C (1975) Lymphoid tumours of the orbit. Mod Probl Ophthalmol 14: 361–363

270. Hecht HL, Hollenberg GM, Pradhan AR (1979) Glucagon-induced small intestine hypotonia demonstrating bleeding lymphoma. Gastrointest Radiol 4: 61–63

271. Heelan RT, Filippa DA (1981) Lymphoma of kidney mimicking simple renal cyst on ultrasound. Clin Bull 11: 139–141

272. Heiken JP, Palmer Gold R, Schnur MJ, King DL, Bashist B, Glazer HS (1983) Computed tomography of renal lymphoma with ultrasound correlation. J Comput Assist Tomogr 7: 245–250

273. Henderson JN (1973) Orbital tumors. Saunders, Philadelphia

274. Henderson JW, Farrow GM (1980) Primary malignant mixed tumors of the lacrimal gland. Ophthalmology 87: 473–475

275. Heni N, Heilmann HP (1971) Magenbefall bei Lymphogranulomatose. Radiologe 11: 356–359

276. Hennessey JP (1958) Discussion of paper by Hahn G: Gynecologic considerations in malignant lymphoma. Am J Obstet Gynecol 75: 673–783

277. Herrmann R, Panahon AM, Barcos MP, Walsh D, Stutzman L (1980) Gastrointestinal involvement in non-Hodgkin's lymphoma. Cancer 46: 215–222

278. Hery M, Dujardin P, Chauvel P, Heldt JP, Namer M (1980) Maladie de Hodgkin. Calcifications ganglionnaires médiastinales après radiothérapie. Bull Cancer (Paris) 67: 337–340

279. Hery M, Thyss A, Boublil JL, Lesbats G, Namer M, Schneider M (1982) Lymphosarcomes primitifs du sein. Quatre observations. Nouv Presse Med 11: 1011

280. Hertz M, Solomon A, Aghai E (1977) "Ivory vertebra" in Hodgkin's disease. Restoration of trabecular pattern after therapy. JAMA 238: 2402

281. Hessel SJ, Adams DF, Abrams HL (1977) Lymphography in lymphoma. In: Clouse ME (ed) Clinical lymphography. Williams and Wilkins, Baltimore, pp 160–184

282. Hietala SO, Wahlqvist L (1982) Metastatic tumors to the kidney. A postmortem, radiologic and clinical investigation. Acta Radiol [Diagn] 23: 585–591

283. Hildell J, Nyman U, Rosengren JE (1981) Lymphoma of the colon detected by CT. Br J Radiol 54: 144–146

284. Hillman BJ, Haber K (1980) Echographic characteristics of malignant lymph nodes. J Clin Ultrasound 8: 213–215

285. Hilweg D, Novak D (1971) Röntgensymptomatik und Häufigkeit einer Magenmanifestation maligner Lymphome. Z Gastroenterol 9: 277–284

286. Hilweg D, Novak D (1972) Röntgenologische Symptomatik einer Dünn- und Dickdarm-Manifestation maligner Lymphome. Z Gastroenterol 10: 315–324

287. Hoerni B, Leleu JP, Durand M, Chauvergne J (1973) Localisations hépatiques de la maladie de Hodgkin. Circonstances de survenue. Med Chir Dig 2: 337–336

288. Hoerr SO, Mac Cormack LJ, Hertzer NR (1973) Prognosis in gastric lymphoma. Arch Surg 107: 155–158

289. Hoffken K, Hornung G, Becker G, Schmidt CG (1973) Die gastrointestinale Manifestation des Morbus Hodgkin. Med Welt 24: 731–732

290. Hope-Stone HF (1979) The diagnosis of osteonecrosis in Hodgkin's disease. Active disease or infarction? Br J Radiol 52: 580–582

291. Horten B, Price RW, Jimenez D (1981) Multifocal varicella-zoster virus leukoencephalitis temporally remote from herpes zoster. Ann Neurol 9: 251–266

292. Hricak H, Thoeni RF, Margulis AR, Eyler WR, Francis IR (1980) Extension of gastric lymphoma into the oesophagus and duodenum. Radiology 135: 309–312

293. Huberman MS, Bunn PA Jr, Matthews MJ, Ihde DC, Gazdar AT, Cohen MH, Minna JD (1980) Hepatic involvement in the cutaneous T-cell lymphomas. Results of percutaneous biopsy and peritoneoscopy. Cancer 45: 1683–1688

294. Hugues FC, Isal JP, Marche J (1974) Les sarcomes lymphocytiques et lymphoblastiques primitifs du poumon. Poumon et Coeur 30: 325–338

295. Hustu HO, Pinkel D (1967) Lymphosarcoma, Hodgkin's disease and leukemia in bone. Clin Orthop 52: 83–93

296. Ichiya Y, Oshiumi Y, Kamoi I, Imoto T, Shimoda Y, Kitagawa S, Matsuura K (1982) 67 Ga scanning and upper gastrointestinal series for gastric lymphomas. Radiology 142: 187–192

297. Irvine RA, Robertson WB (1964) Spinal cord compression in malignant lymphomas. Br Med J 1: 1354–1356

298. Isaacson P, Wright DH (1978) Intestinal lymphoma associated with malabsorption. Lancet 1: 67–70

299. Isaacson P, Wright DH, Judd MA, Mepham BC (1979) Primary gastrointestinal lymphomas. A classification of 66 cases. Cancer 43: 1805-1819

300. Israel RH (1977) Mycosis fungoïdes with rapidly progressive pulmonary infiltration. Radiology 125: 10

301. Jacobs DS (1963) Primary gastric malignant lymphoma and pseudolymphoma. Am J Clin Pathol 40: 379-394

302. Jacobs E, Brombart JC, Cauche C, Pallet P (1971) Aspect radiologique des lymphomes rectocoliques. J Belge Radiol 54: 31-36

303. Jaffe ES, Shevach EM, Frank MM, Berard CW, Green I (1974) Nodular lymphoma. Evidence for origin from follicular lymphocytes. N Engl J Med 290: 813-819

304. Jaffe ES, Berard CW (1978) Lymphoblastic lymphoma, a term rekindled with new precision. Ann Intern Med 89: 415-417

305. Jafri SZH, Bree RL, Amendola MA, Glazer GM, Schwab RE, Francis IR, Borlaza G (1982) CT of renal and perirenal non-Hodgkin lymphoma. Am J Roentgenol 138: 1101-1105

306. Jafri SZH, Francis IR, Glazer GM, Bree RL, Amendola MA (1983) CT detection of adrenal lymphoma. J Comput Assist Tomogr 7: 254-256

307. Jakobiec FA, Mac Lean I, Font R (1979) Clinicopathologic characteristics of orbital lymphoid hyperplasia. Ophthalmology 86: 948-966

308. Jakobiec FA, Henkind P (1980) Ophthalmic CT scanner. The quest for precision and specificity. Ophthalmology 87: 13

309. Jakobiec FA, Gibraltar RA, Knowles DM II, Iwamoto T (1980) Lymphoid tumor of the lid. Ophthalmology 87: 1058-1064

310. Jazy FK, Shehata WM, Tew JM, Meyer RL, Boss HH (1980) Primary intracranial lymphoma of the dura. Arch Neurol 37: 528-529

311. Jenkins PF, Ward MJ, Davies P, Fletcher J (1981) Non-Hodgkin's lymphoma, chronic lymphatic leukaemia and the lung. Br J Dis Chest 75: 22-30

312. Jochelson MS, Balikian JP, Mauch P, Liebman H (1983) Peri- and paracardial involvement in lymphoma: a radiographic study of 11 cases. Am J Roentgenol 140: 483-488

313. Johnson CE, Soule EH (1957) Malignant lymphomas as a gynecologic problem: report of 5 cases including one primary lymphosarcoma of the cervix uteri. Obstet Gynecol 9: 149-157

314. Johnson RE, Thomas LB, Johnson SK, Johnston GS (1974) Correlation between abnormal baseline liver tests and long-term clinical course in Hodgkin's disease. Cancer 33: 1123-1126

315. Johnston GS, Go MF, Benua RS, Larson SM, Andrews GA, Hubner KF (1977) Gallium-67 citrate imaging in Hodgkin's disease: final report of cooperative group. J Nucl Med 18: 692-698

316. Jones SE, Bull M, Kadin ME, Dorfman RF, Kaplan HS, Rosenberg SA, Kim H (1973) Non-Hodgkin's lymphomas. IV. Clinicopathologic correlation in 405 cases. Cancer 31: 806-823

317. Jones SE, Fuks Z, Bull M, Kadin ME, Dorfman RF, Kaplan HS, Rosenberg SA, Kim H (1973) Non-Hodgkin's lymphomas. IV. Clinicopathologic correlation in 405 cases. Cancer 31: 806-823

318. Jones SE, Fuks Z, Kaplan HS, Rosenberg SA (1973) Non-Hodgkin's lymphomas. V. Results of radiotherapy. Cancer 32: 682-691

319. Jones SE, Tobias DA, Waldman RS (1978) Computed tomographic scanning in patients with lymphoma. Cancer 41: 480-486

320. Jonsson K, Lunderquist A (1974) Angiography of the liver and spleen in Hodgkin's disease. Am J Roentgenol 121: 789-792

321. Joseph JI, Lattes R (1966) Gastric lymphosarcoma. Clinicopathologic analysis of 71 cases and its relation to disseminated lymphosarcoma. Am J Clin Pathol 45: 653-669

322. Jucker C, Babini L (1962) La radioterapia dei tumori maligni della tonsilla. Radiol Radioter Fis Med 17: 350-362

323. Kademian MT, Wirtanen GW (1977) Accuracy of bipedal lymphography in Hodgkin's disease. Am J Roentgenol 129: 1041-1042

324. Kadin ME, Glatstein E, Dorfman RF (1971) Clinicopathologic studies of 117 untreated patients subjected to laparotomy for the staging of Hodgkin's disease. Cancer 27: 1281-1294

325. Kahn LB, Selzer G, Kaschula ROC (1972) Primary gastrointestinal lymphoma. A clinicopathologic study of fifty-seven cases. Am J Dig Dis 17: 219-232

326. Kanfer A, Vandewalle A, Maroger LM, Feinterch MJ, Sraer JD, Roland J (1976) Acute renal insufficiency due to lymphomatous infiltration of the kidneys. Cancer 38: 2588-2592

327. Kantor G, Cosset JM, Masselot J (1982) Intérêts de la scanographie thoracique pour le traitement des lymphomes à localisation médiastinale. Bull Cancer 69: 221-225

328. Kaplan HS (1968) Prognostic significance of the relapse-free interval after radiotherapy in Hodgkin's disease. Cancer 22: 1131-1136

329. Kaplan HS (1971) Contiguity and progression in Hodgkin's disease. Cancer Res 31: 1811-1813

330. Kaplan HS (1980) Hodgkin's disease, 2nd edn. Harvard University Press, Cambridge

331. Kaplan J, Mastrangelo R, Peterson WD (1974) Childhood lymphoblastic lymphoma, a cancer of thymus derived lymphocytes. Cancer Res 34: 521-525

332. Katz M, Piekarski P, Bayle-Weisgerber C, Laval-Jeantet M, Teillet F (1977) Masses médiastinales résiduelles post-radiothérapiques au cours de la maladie de Hodgkin. Ann Radiol 20: 667-672

333. Katz M, Laval-Jeantet M (1978) Manifestations intrathoraciques des hémopathies. In: Bismuth V, Blery M, Remy J, Bernadac P, Coulomb M

(eds) Traité de radiodiagnostic, vol IV-2. Masson, Paris, pp 291–303

334. Katz PB, Lee YY, Wallace S, Ray RD (1981) Myelography of spinal block from epidural tumor. AJNR 2: 121–123

335. Kaude JV, Joyce PH (1980) Evaluation of abdominal lymphoma by ultrasound. Gastrointest Radiol 5: 249–254

336. Kazner E, Wilske J, Steinhoff H, Stochdorph O (1978) Computer assisted tomography in primary malignant lymphomas of the brain. J Comput Assist Tomogr 2: 125–134

337. Kenyon R, Ackerman LV (1955) Malignant lymphoma of the thyroid apparently arising in struma lymphomatosa. Cancer 8: 964–969

338. Kern WH, Crepfan AG, Jones JC (1961) Primary Hodgkin's disease of the lung. Report of four cases and review of the literature. Cancer 14: 1151–1165

339. Kevers L, Brucher JM, Laterre EC (1980) Image tomodensitométrique en miroir dans un cas de lymphome malin du cerveau. Acta Neurol Belg 80: 86–94

340. Kielly JM, Massey BD, Harrison EG, Utz DC (1970) Lymphoma of the testis. Cancer 26: 847–852

341. Kim H, Dorfman RF, Rosenberg SA (1976) Pathology of malignant lymphomas in the liver: application in staging. Prog Liver Dis 5: 683–698

342. Kinsella TJ, Glatstein E (1983) Staging laparotomy and splenectomy for Hodgkin's disease: current status. Cancer Investigation 1: 87–91

343. Kirsch J, Rosenthal L, Finlayson MH, Wee R (1976) Progressive multifocal leukoencephalopathy. Radiology 119: 399–400

344. Kline TS, Goldstein F (1973) Malignant lymphoma involving the stomach. Cancer 32: 961–968

345. Knowles DM II, Jakobiec FA (1980) Orbital lymphoid neoplasms. A clinicopathologic study of 60 patients. Cancer 46: 576–589

346. Kobayashi T, Takatani O, Kimura K (1976) Echographic patterns of malignant lymphoma. J Clin Ultrasound 4: 181–186

347. Koehler PR (1978) Lymphography vs CT of lymphomas. Am J Roentgenol 131: 1116–1117

348. Kolaric K, Roth A, Dominis M, Jakasa V (1977) The diagnostic value of percutaneous liver biopsy in patients with non Hodgkin's lymphoma. A preliminary report. Acta Hepato-Gastroenterol 24: 440–443

349. Kolygin BA, Vesnin AG (1976) Hodgkin's disease in children. Clinico-roentgenologic features of the lesion in the chest. Pediat Radiol 4: 144–148

350. Kretzchmar K, Guttahr P, Kutzner J (1980) CT studies before and after CNS treatment for acute lymphoblastic leukemia and malignant non-Hodgkin's lymphoma in childhood. Neuroradiology 20: 173–180

351. Krolikiewicz H, Maruyama Y, De Land H, Beihn RM, Hafner TV, Kim EE (1978) 67 Gasubtraction scanning in Hodgkin's disease and lymphomas. Acta Radiol Oncol 17: 296–304

352. Krudy AG, Dunnick NR, Magrath IT, Shawker TH, Doppman JL, Spiegel R (1981) CT of American Burkitt lymphoma. Am J Roentgenol 136: 747–754

353. Kushelev AE (1975) Lymphogranulomatosis of the caecum. Vrach Delo 10: 99–100

354. Kyaw M, Koehler PR (1969) Renal and perirenal lymphoma: arteriographic findings. Radiology 93: 1055–1058

355. Lacher MJ (1983) Routine staging laparotomy for patients with Hodgkin's disease is no longer necessary. Cancer Invest 1: 93–99

356. Lalande C, Dulac O, Marvault C, Bennet J (1980) Accident vasculaire cérébral après traitement prophylactique sur le système nerveux central des leucémies aigues lymphoblastiques et lymphomes. Ann Radiol 23: 81–86

357. Lalli AF (1969) Lymphoma and the urinary tract. Radiology 93: 1051–1054

358. Lamarque JL, Ginestie JF, Combes C (1968) Valeur de la lymphographie dans le diagnostic précoce des adénopathies rétropéritonéales (bilan de 450 explorations). Ann Radiol 11: 888–893

359. Lasala FG, Lopez H, Dadoni LRAG, Sagasta CL (1970) Enfermedad de Hodgkin con localizacion en el intestino grueso. Prensa Med Argent 57: 109–114

360. Lathrop JC (1967) Views and reviews: malignant pelvic lymphomas. Obstet Gynecol 30: 137–145

361. Laurin S (1975) Cavography and lymphography in Hodgkin's disease. Acta Radiol [Diagn] 16: 98–106

362. Le Bourgeois JP, Delalande B, Vergnes G, Kuentz M (1983) Irradiation en mantelet dans la maladie de Hodgkin. Influence de la taille du médiastin sur le risque péricardique. Presse Med 12: 772

363. Lecomte P, Bruneton JN, Eloit J, Bourry J, Aubanel D, Schneider M (1980) Manifestations radiologiques des localisations digestives extragastriques des lymphomes non-hodgkiniens. A propos de 25 observations. Ann Gastroenterol Hepatol 16: 463–471

364. Lecomte P, Bruneton JN, Rouison D (1980) Lymphomes malins de l'estomac. J Can Assoc Radiol 31: 101–106

365. Le Cudonnec B, Chermet J, Fragoas M (1975) Aspects radiologiques des lymphoréticulosarcomes gastriques primitifs. A propos de 20 cas. Ann Radiol (Paris) 18: 609–618

366. Lee CKK, Bloomfield CD, Goldman AI, Levitt SH (1980) Prognostic significance of mediastinal involvement in Hodgkin's disease treated with curative radiotherapy. Cancer 46: 2403–2409

367. Lee KR, Levine E, Moffat RE, Bigongiari LR, Hermeck AS (1979) Computed tomographic staging of malignant gastric neoplasms. Radiology 133: 151-155

368. Lee JKT, Stanley RJ, Sagel SS, Melson GL, Koehler RE (1980) Limitations of the post-lymphangiogram plain abdominal radiograph as an indicator of recurrent lymphoma. Comparison to computed tomography. Radiology 134: 155-158

369. Léger L, Chiche B, Louvel A, Bertin J (1979) Sarcomes lymphoides primitifs de l'estomac. Nouv Presse Med 8: 99-103

370. Lehrer S, Roswit B (1978) Primary lymphoma of the paranasal sinuses. Ann Otol Rhinol Laryngol 87: 81-84

371. Lennert K, Mohri N, Stein H, Kaiserling E (1975) The histopathology of malignant lymphoma. Br J Haematol 31 [Suppl]: 193-203

372. Lenzi P, Molinari R (1967) I: Reticulosarcomi della base linguale. Ann Laring 66: 957-978

373. Lepage E, Ferme C, Frija J, Gayet B, Clot P, D'Agay MF, Gisselbrecht C, Marty M, Boiron M (1984) Maladie de Hodgkin. Masses résiduelles histologiquement non évolutives après chimiothérapie. Presse Med 13: 1766-1769

374. Levin DC, Gordon DH, Kinkhabwala M, Becker JA (1976) Arteriography of retroperitoneal lymphoma. Am J Roentgenol 126: 368-375

375. Levitan R, Diamond HD, Craver LF (1971) The liver in Hodgkin's disease. Gut 2: 60-71

376. Levitt LJ, Ainsenberg AC, Harris NL, Linggood RM, Poppema S (1982) Primary non-Hodgkin's lymphoma of the mediastinum. Cancer 50: 2486-2492

377. Lewin KJ, Ranchod M, Dorfman RF (1978) Lymphomas of the gastrointestinal tract. A study of 117 cases presenting with gastrointestinal disease. Cancer 42: 693-707

378. Lewis E, Bernardino ME, Salvador PG, Cabanillas FF, Barnes PA, Thomas JL (1982) Post-therapy CT-detected mass in lymphoma patients: is it viable tissue? J Comput Assist Tomogr 6: 792-795

379. Libshitz HI, Banner MP (1974) Spontaneous pneumothorax as a complication of radiation therapy of the thorax. Radiology 112: 199-201

380. Libshitz HI, Green B (1979) Kidney. In: Libshitz HI (ed) Diagnostic radiology of radiotherapy change. Williams and Wilkins, Baltimore, pp 111-122

381. Libshitz HI, Jonsson K (1979) Lymphatic system. In: Libshitz HI (ed) Diagnostic roentgenology of radiotherapy change. Williams and Wilkins, Baltimore, pp 185-194

382. Libshitz HI, Shumann LS (1984) Radiation-induced pulmonary changes: CT findings. J Comput Assist Tomogr 8: 15-19

383. Libshitz HI, Southard ME (1974) Complications of radiation therapy: the thorax. Sem Roentgenol 9: 41-49

384. Libshitz HI, Brosof AB, Southard ME (1973) Radiographic appearance of the chest following extended field radiation therapy for Hodgkin's disease. A consideration of the time-dose relationships. Cancer 32: 203-215

385. Libshitz HI, Zornoza J, Mc Larty JW (1978) Lung cancer in chronic leukemia and lymphoma. Radiology 127: 297-300

386. Lichtenstein AK, Levine A, Taylor CR, Boswell W, Rossman S, Feinstein DI, Lukes RJ (1980) Primary lymphoma in adults. Am J Med 68: 509-514

387. Lobe LP, Katenkamp D (1981) Zur Klinik und Therapie maligner non-Hodgkin Lymphome der Nasennebenhöhlenregion. Laryngol Rhinol Otol 60: 334-337

388. Lochridge SK, Knibbe WP, Doty DB (1979) Obstruction of the superior vena cava. Surgery 85: 14-24

389. Loehr WJ, Mujahed Z, Zahn FD, Gray GF, Thorbjarnarson B (1969) Primary lymphoma of the gastrointestinal tract: a review of 100 cases. Ann Surg 170: 232-238

390. Lopez-Majano V, Sion A, Friedell MT, Chefec G, Abraira C (1975) Subacute thyroiditis associated with lymphosarcoma of the thyroid. Int Surg 60: 172-176

391. Lucia SP, Mills H, Lowenhaupt E, Hunt ML (1952) Visceral involvement in primary neoplastic diseases of the reticuloendothelial system. Cancer 5: 1193-1200

392. Lucke B, Schlumberger HG (1957) Tumors of the kidney, renal pelvis and ureter. Atlas of tumor pathology, Fasc 30. AFIP, Washington

393. Lukes RJ (1971) Criteria for involvement of lymph nodes, bone marrow, spleen and liver in Hodgkin's disease. Cancer Res 31: 1755-1767

394. Lukes RJ, Butler JJ (1966) The pathology and nomenclature of Hodgkin's disease. Cancer Res 26: 1063-1081

395. Lukes RJ, Collins RD (1974) Immunological characterization of human malignant lymphomas. Cancer 34: 1488-1503

396. Lunderquist A, Lunderquist A, Holmdahl KH, Clemens F (1971) Selective superior mesenteric arteriography in reticular-cell sarcoma of the small bowel. Radiology 98: 113-115

397. Macdonald JS, Peckham MJ (1973) Lymphography. In: Smithers D (ed) Hodgkin's disease. Churchill Livingstone, Edinburgh, pp 169-178

398. Macht SD, Pett SD, Tsangaris NT (1979) Non-Hodgkin lymphoma of the parotid gland: diagnosis, evaluation, and treatment. Ann Plast Surg 2: 37-41

399. MacInerney DP, Bullimore J (1977) Reactivation of radiation pneumonitis by adriamycin. Br J Radiol 50: 224-227

400. Macintosh PK, Thomson KR, Barbaric LL (1979) Percutaneous transperitoneal lymph-node biopsy as a means of improving lymphographic diagnosis. Radiology 131: 647-649

401. MacLennan TW, Castellino RA (1975) Calcification in pelvic lymph nodes containing Hodgkin's disease following radiotherapy. Radiology 115: 87–89

402. MacNeer G, Berg JW (1959) The clinical behavior and management of primary malignant lymphoma of the stomach. Surgery 46: 829–840

403. MacNelis FL, Pai VT (1969) Malignant lymphoma of head and neck. Laryngoscope 79: 1076–1087

404. Maeda M, Kotake Y, Mondeau Y, Nakahara K, Kawashima Y, Kitamura H (1981) Primary lymphoma of the trachea: report of a case treated by primary end-to-end anastomosis after circumferential resection of the trachea. J Thorac Cardiovasc Surg 81: 835–839

405. Magnusson A, Hagberg H, Hemmingsson A, Lindgren PG (1982) Computed tomography, ultrasound and lymphography in the diagnosis of malignant lymphoma. Acta Radiol [Diagn] 23: 29–35

406. Makinen J, Alfthan O, Vuori J (1979) Malignant lymphoma of the urinary bladder. A report of 2 cases. Eur Urol 5: 45–57

407. Mambo NC, Burke JS, Butler JJ (1977) Primary malignant lymphomas of the breast. Cancer 39: 2033–2040

408. Mancuso AA, Hanafee WN (1982) Computed tomography of the head and neck. Williams and Wilkins, Baltimore

409. Mancuso AA, Maceri D, Rice D, Hanafee WN (1981) CT of cervical lymph node cancer. Am J Roentgenol 136: 381–385

410. Mandell GA, Lantieri R, Goodman LR (1982) Tracheobronchial compression in Hodgkin lymphoma in children. Am J Roentgenol 139: 1167–1170

411. Marcuse PM, Stout AP (1950) Primary lymphosarcoma of small intestine: analysis of 13 cases and review of literature. Cancer 3: 459–474

412. Margineanu N (1963) Aspecte radiologice ale leziunilor tubuliu digestiv in boala Hodgkin. Oncol Radiol 2: 261–265

413. Marglin SI, Castellino RA (1981) Lymphographic accuracy in 632 consecutive, previously untreated cases of Hodgkin disease and non-Hodgkin lymphoma. Radiology 40: 341–353

414. Marglin SI, Soulen RL, Blank N, Castellino RA (1979) Mycosis fungoides. Radiographic manifestations of extracutaneous intrathoracic involvement. Radiology 130: 35–37

415. Mark LK (1977) Primary lymphoma of the lung. JAMA 237: 895–896

416. Markiewicz W, Glatstein E, London EJ, Popp RL (1977) Echocardiographic detection of pericardial effusion and pericardial thickening in malignant lymphoma. Radiology 123: 161–164

417. Markovits P, Bergiron C, Guinard J, Contesso G (1975) Etude radioclinique des localisations mammaires des hématosarcomes. Ann Radiol 18: 711–720

418. Marshak RH, Lindner AE, Maklansky D (1976) Lymphosarcoma of the stomach. Am J Gastroenterol 66: 176–184

419. Marshak RH, Lindner AE, Maklansky D (1976) Immunoglobulin disorders of the small bowel. Radiol Clin North Am 14: 477–491

420. Marshak RH, Lindner AE, Maklansky D (1979) Lymphoreticular disorders of the gastrointestinal tract: roentgenographic features. Gastrointest Radiol 4: 103–120

421. Marshall SF, Adamson NE Jr (1959) Malignant tumors of stomach. Surg Clin North Am 39: 699–701

422. Marshall SF, Adamson NE Jr (1959) Sarcoma of the stomach. Tumors of lymphatic and reticuloendothelial origin (62 cases). Surg Clin North Am 39: 711–718

423. Martinez-Maldonado M, Ramirez de Arellano GA (1966) Renal involvement in malignant lymphomas. A survey of 49 cases. J Urol 95: 485–488

424. Mathe G, Rappaport H, O'Connor GT, Torloni H (1976) Histological and cytological typing of neoplastic diseases of hematopoetic and lymphoid tissues. In: WHO International histological classification of tumours, no 14. WHO, Geneva

425. Mattingly SS, Cibull ML, Ram MD, Hagihara PF, Griffen WO (1981) Pseudolymphoma of the stomach. A diagnostic and therapeutic dilemma. Arch Surg 116: 25–29

426. Mauch P, Goodman R, Hellman S (1978) The significance of mediastinal involvement in early Hodgkin's disease. Cancer 42: 1039–1045

427. Mehrotra RML, Wahal KM, Agrawal PK (1979) Testicular lymphoma: a clinicopathologic study of 22 cases. Indian J Pathol Microbiol 22: 301–305

428. M. nuck LS (1976) Gastric lymphoma, a radiologic diagnosis. Gastrointest Radiol 1: 157–161

429. Merill J, Greco FA, Zimbler A, Brereton HD, Lamberg JD, Pomeroy TC (1975) Adriamycin and radiation: synergistic cardiotoxicity. Ann Inter Med 82: 122–123

430. Meyer JE, Kopans B, Long JC (1980) Mammographic appearance of malignant lymphoma of the breast. Radiology 135: 623–626

431. Meyers MA, Katzen B, Alonso DR (1975) Transpyloric extension to duodenal bulb in gastric lymphoma. Radiology 115: 575–580

432. Mikal S (1964) Primary lymphoma of the thyroid gland. Surgery 55: 233–239

433. Milder MS, Larson SM, Bagley CM Jr, De Vita VT Jr, Johnson RE, Johnston GS (1973) Liverspleen scan in Hodgkin's disease. Cancer 31: 826–834

434. Miller JB, Variakojis D, Bitran JD, Sweet DL Jr, Golomb HM, Ultmann JE (1981) Diffuse histiocytic lymphoma with sclerosis: a clinicopathologic entity frequently causing superior vena caval obstruction. Cancer 47: 748–756

435. Miller JH, Hindman BW, Lam AHK (1980) Ultrasound in the evaluation of small bowel lymphoma in children. Radiology 135: 409-414

436. Mirra JM (1980) Bone tumors, diagnosis and treatment. Lippincott, Philadelphia

437. Modan B, Shani M, Goldman B, Modan M (1969) Nodal and extranodal malignant lymphoma in Israel: an epidemiological study. Br J Hematol 16: 53-59

438. Monohan DJ (1965) Hodgkin's disease of the lung. J Thor Cardiovasc Surg 49: 173-175

439. Morrison FS, Critz F, Tatum WT, Stauss HK (1973) Hodgkin's disease of the esophagus: successful treatment of a rare complication. Cancer 31: 1244-1246

440. Moss AA, Schrumpf J, Schnyder P, Korobkin M, Shimshak RR (1979) Computed tomography of focal hepatic lesions: a blind clinical evaluation of the effect of contrast enhancement. Radiology 131: 427-430

441. Mould JJ, Adam NM (1983) The problem of avascular necrosis of bone in patients treated for Hodgkin's disease. Clin Radiol 34: 231-236

442. Mueller PR, Ferrucci JT Jr, Harbin WP, Kirkpatrick RH, Simeone JF, Wittenberg J (1980) Appearance of lymphomatous involvement of the mesentery by ultrasonography and body computed tomography: the "sandwich sign". Radiology 134: 467-473

443. Murphy WT, Bilge N (1964) Compression of the spinal cord in patients with malignant lymphoma. Radiology 82: 495-501

444. Musshoff K (1971) Prognostic and therapeutic implications of staging in extranodal Hodgkin's disease. Cancer Res 31: 1814-1827

445. Musshoff K (1977) Klinische Stadieneinteilung der Nicht-Hodgkin-Lymphome. Strahlentherapie 153: 218-221

446. Najman A, Gorin NC, Barranger C, Duhamel G (1977) Les localisations digestives des lymphomes non-hodgkiniens. 31 cas. Nouv Presse Med 6: 3515-3519

447. Nakada T, St John JN, Knight RJ (1983) Solitary metastasis of systemic malignant lymphoma to the cerebellopontine angle. Neuroradiology 24: 225-228

448. Naqvi MS, Burrows L, Kark AE (1969) Lymphoma of the gastrointestinal tract. Prognostic guides based on 162 cases. Ann Surg 170: 221-231

449. Nassar VH, Salem PA, Shadid MJ, Alami SY, Balikian JB, Salem AA, Nasrallah SM (1978) "Mediterranean abdominal lymphoma" or immunoproliferative small intestinal disease. Part II: pathological aspects. Cancer 41: 1340-1354

450. Nathwani BN, Kim H, Rappaport H (1976) Malignant lymphoma, lymphoblastic. Cancer 38: 964-983

451. Nathwani BN, Diamond LW, Winberg CD, Kim H, Bearman RM, Glick JH, Jones SE, Gams RA, Nissen NI, Rappaport H (1981) Lymphoblastic lymphoma: a clinicopathologic study of 95 patients. Cancer 48: 2347-2357

452. Negrin-Fragoas M, Taieb A, Chermet J, Bigot JM, Monnier JP (1975) Etude anatomoclinique et radiologique des lymphoréticulosarcomes coliques. A propos de 8 observations. J Radiol 56: 49-60

453. Neiman HL, Goldstein HM, Silverman PJ, Bookstein JJ (1975) Angiographic features of peripancreatic malignant lymphoma. Radiology 115: 589-592

454. Nelson DF, Reddy V, O'Mara RE, Rubin P (1978) Thyroid abnormalities following neck irradiation for Hodgkin's disease. Cancer 42: 2553-2562

455. Nelson GA, Dockerty MB, Pratt JH, Remine WH (1958) Malignant lymphoma involving the ovaries. Am J Obstet Gynecol 76: 861-871

456. Nenoff RS, Young SW, Noon MA, Castellino RA (1981) CT appearance of renal lymphomas. 67th annual meeting of the Radiological Society of North America, Chicago

457. Neumann CH, Robert NJ, Canellos G, Rosenthal D (1983) Computed tomography of the abdomen and pelvis in non-Hodgkin lymphoma. J Comput Assist Tomogr 7: 846-850

458. Neumann CH, Robert NJ, Rosenthal D, Canellos G (1983) Clinical value of ultrasonography for the management of non-Hodgkin lymphoma patients as compared with abdominal tomography. J Comput Assist Tomogr 7: 666-669

459. New GB, Stevenson W (1943) End results of malignant lesions of the nasopharynx. AMA Arch Otolaryng 38: 205-209

460. Ngan H, Preston BJ (1975) Non-Hodgkin's lymphoma presenting with osseous lesions. Clin Radiol 26: 351-356

461. Nguyen GK (1982) Primary extranodal non-Hodgkin's lymphoma of the extrahepatic bile ducts. Report of a case. Cancer 50: 2218-2222

462. Niblett JS (1975) Forty-year survival in Hodgkin's disease with calcified lymph nodes. Br J Radiol 48: 396

463. Nicoloff DM, Haynes LB, Wangensteen OH (1963) Primary lymphosarcoma of the gastrointestinal tract. Surg Gynecol Obstet 117: 433-437

464. Nime FA, Cooper HS, Eggleston JC (1976) Primary malignant lymphomas of the salivary glands. Cancer 37: 906-912

465. Nissan S, Bar-Moar JA, Levy C (1974) Lymphosarcoma of the esophagus: a case report. Cancer 34: 1321-1323

466. Nobrega FT, Kyle RA, Harrison EG Jr (1973) Malignant lymphoma including Hodgkin's disease occurring in the vicinity of a large medical center (Olmsted County, Minn, 1945 through 1969). Cancer 31: 295-302

467. Noon MA, Brant-Zawadzki M, Young SW, Castellino RA (1979) Radiographic findings of lym-

phoma involving the larynx: a report of two cases. Am J Roentgenol 132: 457-458

468. Norfray J, Calenoff L, Zanon B Jr (1973) Aneurismal lymphoma of the small intestine. Am J Roentgenol 119: 335-341

469. North LB, Fuller LM, Hagemeister FB, Rodgers RW, Butler JJ, Shurlemberger CC (1982) Importance of initial mediastinal adenopathy in Hodgkin disease. Am J Roentgenol 138: 229-235

470. Novak D, Probst P (1973) Morbus Hodgkin: Häufigkeit und Lokalisation der Lungen-, Knochen- und Magen-Darm-manifestation. Strahlentherapie 146: 403-413

471. Novak S, Caraveo J, Trowbridge AA, Peterson RF, White RR III (1979) Primary lymphomas of the gastrointestinal tract. South Med J 72: 1154-1158

472. O'Connell DJ, Thompson AJ (1978) Lymphoma of the colon: the spectrum of radiologic changes. Gastrointest Radiol 2: 377-385

473. O'Conor GT (1961) Malignant lymphoma in African children. II. A pathological entity. Cancer 14: 270-283

474. Okamato M, Ushio Y, Kinoshita A (1973) Roentgenologic diagnosis of gastrointestinal malignant lymphomas. Stomach Intest (Tokyo) 8: 149-163

475. Okuno T, Carstens HP (1973) Perforated jejunum due to primary Hodgkin's disease. Ill Med J 143: 343-344

476. Olumide AA, Osunkoya BO, Ngu VA (1971) Superior mediastinal compression: a report of five cases caused by malignant lymphoma. Cancer 27: 193-202

477. Ornstein DH, Ruoff M (1977) The radiology corner. Hodgkin's disease of the small intestine. Am J Gastroenterol 68: 182-187

478. Osteaux M, Dewilde A, Jeanmart L, Bollaert A (1975) Apport de la lymphographie au diagnostic différentiel des lymphomes malins. J Belge Radiol 56: 399-406

479. Pagani JJ, Bernardino ME (1981) CT Radiographic correlation of ulcerating small bowel lymphomas. Am J Roentgenol 136: 998-1000

480. Pagani JJ, Libshitz HI (1982) CT manifestations of radiation induced change in chest tissue. J Comput Assist Tomogr 6: 243-248

481. Pagani JJ, Libshitz MI, Wallace S, Hayman LA (1981) CNS leukemia and lymphoma: CT manifestations. AJNR 2: 397-403

482. Pagatlunan RJG, Mayo CW, Dockerty MB (1964) Primary malignant tumors of the small intestine. Am J Surg 108: 13-18

483. Palacios E, Gorelick PB, Gonzalez CF, Fine M (1982) Malignant lymphoma of the nervous system. J Comput Assist Tomogr 6: 689-701

484. Papaionnou AN, Watsun WL (1965) Primary lymphoma of the lung: appraisal of its natural history and comparison with other localised

lymphoma. J Thorac Cardiovasc Surg 49: 373-387

485. Parker BR, Blank N, Castellino RA (1974) Lymphographic appearance of benign conditions simulating lymphoma. Radiology 111: 267-274

486. Parker BR, Castellino RA, Kaplan SA (1976) Pediatric Hodgkin's disease. I. Radiographic evaluation. Cancer 37: 2430-2435

487. Patchefsky AS, Brodovsky HS, Menduke H, Southard M, Brooks J, Nicklas D, Hoch WS (1974) Non-Hodgkin's lymphomas: a clinicopathologic study of 293 cases. Cancer 34: 1173-1186

488. Paulet P, Cauchie C, Jacobs E (1969) Lymphomes malins avec entreprise rectale. Trois cas dont une maladie de Brill-Symmers à point de départ rectosigmoïdien. Acta Gastroenterol Belg 32: 684-693

489. Pear BL (1974) Skeletal manifestations of the lymphomas and leukemia. Sem Roentgenol 9: 229-240

490. Peckhamm D (1973) Lung involvement. In: Smithers D (ed) Hodgkin's disease. Churchill Livingstone, Edinburgh, pp 118-127

491. Peeples WJ, El Mahdi AM, Rosato FE (1979) Achalasia of the esophagus associated with Hodgkin disease. J Surg Oncol 11: 213-216

492. Perez CA, Dorfman RF (1966) Benign lymphoid hyperplasia of the stomach and duodenum. Radiology 87: 505-510

493. Perez-Aguilar F, Olaso V, Rivas S, Rodrigo Moreno M, Devesa F, Berenguer J (1980) Linfoma intestinal como complication de la enfermedad celiaca. Rev Clin Esp 157: 53-56

494. Perreau P, Gardais J, Pithon G (1972) Lymphosarcome mammaire primitif bilatéral de la femme jeune. J Gyn Obst Biol Repr 1: 273-280

495. Petterson H, Harwood-Nash DC, Fitz CR, Chuang S, Amstrong E (1981) Contrast enhancement of the irradiated spinal cord in children. AJNR 2: 581-584

496. Petzel H, Mathea H (1972) Ausgedehnte lymphatische Hyperplasie im Magen-Darm-Trakt und Lymphosarkomatose. Fortschr Röntgenstr 116: 523-529

497. Philipps WC, Kattapuran SV, Doseretz DE, Raymond AK, Schiller AL, Murphy G, Wyshak G (1982) Primary lymphoma of bone: relationship of radiographic appearance and prognosis. Radiology 144: 285-290

498. Phillips TL, Margolis LW (1972) Radiation pathology and the clinical response and oesophagus. In: Vaeth JM (ed) Frontiers of radiation therapy and oncology, vol 6. University Park Press, Baltimore, pp 254-273

499. Phillips TL, Wharam MD, Margolis LW (1975) Modification of radiation injury to normal tissues by chemotherapeutic agents. Cancer 35: 1678-1684

500. Pick RA, Castellino RA, Seltzer RA (1971) Arteriographic findings in renal lymphoma. Am J Roentgenol 111: 530-534

501. Pilepitch MV, Rene JB, Munzenrider JE, Carter BL (1978) Contributions of computed tomography to the treatment of lymphoma. Am J Roentgenol 131: 69-73

502. Pinkel D (1975) Non-Hodgkin's lymphoma in children. Br J Cancer 31 [Suppl 2]: 298-323

503. Pochacevsky R, Sherman RS (1962) Diffuse lymphomatous disease of the colon: its roentgen appearance. Am J Roentgenol 87: 670-684

504. Portalez D, Song MY, Marty NH, Joffre F (1982) Ultrasonographic patterns of testicular non-Hodgkin's lymphoma. A report of five cases. Eur J Radiol 2: 222-225

505. Portlock CS, Glatstein E (1978) The non-Hodgkin's lymphomas: current concepts on management. Ann Rev Med 29: 81-89

506. Portlock ES, Rosenberg SA (1979) No initial therapy for stage III and IV non-Hodgkin's lymphomas of favorable histologic types. Ann Intern Med 90: 10-13

507. Portmann UV, Dunne EF, Hazard JB (1954) Manifestations of Hodgkin's disease of the gastrointestinal tract. Am J Roentgenol 72: 772-787

508. Post JD (1980) Radiographic evaluation of the spine. Masson, New York

509. Poujol J (1984) Tumeurs de l'orbite. In: Bruneton JN, Matter D, Benozio M, Senecail B (eds) L'échographie en pathologie tumorale de l'adulte. Masson, Paris, pp 159-164

510. Prakash A, Sharma LK, Koshal A (1974) Primary Hodgkin's disease of the small bowel. Int Surg 59: 488-490

511. Privett JTJ, Rhys Davies E, Roylance J (1977) The radiological features of gastric lymphoma. Clin Radiol 28: 457-463

512. Racek F, Salzman V (1969) Das maligne Lymphogranulom des Dünndarms. Z Ges Inn Med 24: 825-827

513. Radvany J, Levine H (1978) CT in the diagnosis of primary lymphoma of the central nervous system. J Comput Assist Tomogr 2: 215-217

514. Ramos L, Marcos J, Illanas M, Hernandez-Mora M, Perez-Paya F, Picouto JL, Santana P, Chantar C (1978) Radiologic characteristics of primary intestinal lymphoma of the "Mediterranean" type: observations on twelve cases. Radiology 126: 379-385

515. Rappaport H (1966) Tumors of the hematopoietic system. Atlas of tumor pathology, section 3, Fasc 8. AFIP, Washington

516. Rappaport H, Thomas LB (1974) Mycosis fungoïdes: the pathology of extracutaneous involvement. Cancer 34: 1198-1229

517. Rappaport H, Berard CW, Butler JJ, Dorfman RF, Lukes RJ, Thomas LB (1971) Report of the Committee on Histopathological Criteria contributing to staging of Hodgkin's disease. Cancer Res 31: 1864-1865

518. Ravid M, Shapira J, Lang R, Ravid R (1979) Acute respiratory distress syndrome. A presenting symptom of malignant lymphoma. JAMA 241: 2191-2192

519. Read G (1981) Lymphoma of the testis. Results of treatment 1960-77. Clin Radiol 32: 687-692

520. Reimer RR, Chabner BA, Young RC, Reddick R, Johnson RE (1977) Lymphoma presenting in bone. Ann Intern Med 87: 50-56

521. Reunias clinica do ibepege (1979) Colestase extra-hepatica, com obstruçao do colédoco por linfoma histocities. Arq Gastroent S Paolo 16: 100-105

522. Reymond R, Hazra T, El Mahdi AM, Lott S (1971) Primary malignant lymphoma of the bladder. A case report. J Assoc Can Radiol 22: 170-172

523. Richmond J, Sherman RS, Diamond HD, Craver LF (1962) Renal lesions associated with malignant lymphomas. Am J Med 32: 184-207

524. Robb WAT (1978) Lymphoma of the testis. J R Coll Surg Edinb 23: 84-87

525. Roberts WC, Glancy DL, DeVita VT (1968) Heart in malignant lymphoma (Hodgkin's disease, lymphosarcoma, reticulum cell sarcoma and mycosis fungoïdes). A study of 196 autopsy cases. Am J Cardiol 22: 85-107

526. Roesch W, Hartwich G, Moerl M, Fuchs HF (1975) Ungewöhnliche Verlaufsformen maligner Lymphome des Gastro-intestinaltraktes. Leber Magen Darm 5: 239-244

527. Rolf SL, Kratz RC, Tanner GR, Crissman J (1980) Primary lymphoma of the thyroid and Hashimoto's thyroiditis. J Ky Med Assoc 78: 263-266

528. Rosch J (1966) Tumours of the spleen: the value of selective arteriography. Clin Radiol 17: 183-190

529. Rosen PJ, Feinstein DI, Pattengale PK (1978) Convoluted lymphocytic lymphoma in adults: a clinico-pathologic entity. Ann Intern Med 89: 319-324

530. Rosenberg SA (1966) Report of the Committee on the staging of Hodgkin's disease. Cancer Res 25: 1310

531. Rosenberg SA (1971) Hodgkin's disease of the bone marrow. Cancer Res 31: 1733-1736

532. Rosenberg SA (1975) Bone marrow involvement in the non-Hodgkin's lymphomata. Br J Cancer 31 [Suppl 2]: 261-264

533. Rosenberg SA (1977) Validity of the Ann Arbor staging classification for the non Hodgkin's lymphomas. Cancer Treat Rep 61: 1023-1027

534. Rosenberg SA, Diamond HD, Jaslowitz B, Craver LF (1961) Lymphosarcoma: a review of 1269 cases. Medicine 40: 31-84

535. Ross CF, Eley A (1975) Lymphosarcoma of the breast. Br J Surg 62: 651-652

536. Rossi JF, Dubois A, Brunel M, Janbon C, Vallat G (1982) Manifestations rénales de la maladie

de Hodgkin. A propos de deux observations. Revue de la littérature. Sem Hôp Paris 58: 1471-1475

537. Rostock RA, Giangreco A, Wharam MD, Lenhad R, Siegelaman SS, Order SE (1982) CT scan modifications in the treatment of mediastinal Hodgkin's disease. Cancer 49: 2267-2275

538. Rotmensch J, Woodruff JD (1982) Lymphoma of the ovary: report of twenty new cases and update of previous series. Am J Gynecol Obstet 143: 870-875

539. Rottino A, Hoffman G (1955) The pathology of the lung in Hodgkin's disease. Am J Surg 89: 550-555

540. Roze R, Gras F (1965) Le lymphosarcome primitif du caecum. J Radiol 46: 851-854

541. Rubin BE (1979) Computed tomography in the evaluation of renal lymphoma. J Comput Assist Tomogr 3: 759-764

542. Ruckdeschel JC, Chang P, Martin RG, Byhardt RW, O'Connell MJ, Sutherland JC, Wiernick PH (1975) Radiation-related pericardial effusions in patients with Hodgkin's disease. Medicine 54: 245-259

543. Rudders RA, MacCaffrey JA, Kahn PC (1977) The relative roles of Gallium-67-citrate. Scanning and lymphangiography in the current management of malignant lymphoma. Cancer 40: 1439-1443

544. Rudders RA, Ross ME, De Lellis RA (1978) Primary extranodal lymphoma. Response to treatment and factors influencing prognosis. Cancer 42: 406-416

545. Ruppert GB, Smith VM (1979) Multiple lymphomatous polyposis of the gastrointestinal tract. Gastrointest Endosc 25: 67-69

546. Sako M, Kono M, Nishimine M (1979) Lymphographic classification of malignant lymphoma. Lymphology 12: 23-25

547. Salem PA, Nassar VH, Shahid MJ, Hajj AA, Alami SY, Balikian JB, Salem AA (1977) "Mediterranean abdominal lymphoma" or immunoproliferative small intestine disease. Part I: Clinical aspects. Cancer 40: 2941-2947

548. Salem S, Hiltz CW (1978) Ultrasonographic appearance of gastric lymphosarcoma. J Clin Ultrasound 6: 429-430

549. Salmela H, Kohler R (1969) Roentgenological characteristics of mesenchymal tumours of the stomach. Ann Clin Res 1: 57-63

550. Sando I, Black FO, Randolph G, Newell RC (1969) Lymphosarcoma invading the temporal bone contents: a histopathological case report. Laryngoscope 79: 2140-2149

551. Sandusky WR, Jones RCW Jr, Horsley JS, Marsh WL Jr, Tillack TW, Tegtmeyer CJ, Hess CE (1978) Staging laparotomy in Hodgkin's disease. Ann Surg 187: 485-489

552. Schaner EG, Head GL, Doppman JL, Young RC (1977) Computed tomography in the diagnosis, staging and management of abdominal lymphoma. J Comput Assist Tomogr 1: 176-180

553. Scharifker D, Chalasani A (1978) Ureteral involvement by malignant lymphoma: ten years experience. Arch Pathol Lab Med 102: 541-542

554. Schellinger D, Miller WE, Harrison EG Jr, Kiely JM (1974) Lymphographic patterns of the subtypes of malignant lymphoma, including Hodgkin's disease. Radiology 111: 257-266

555. Schey WL, White H, Conway JJ, Kidd JM (1973) Lymphosarcoma in children. A roentgenologic and clinical evaluation of 60 children. Am J Roentgenol 117: 59-72

556. Schmid U, Gloor F, Schildknecht O (1980) Das maligne nicht-Hodgkin-Lymphom des Magens. Dtsch Med Wschr 105: 1147-1152

557. Schneider M, Mathe G, Schwarzenberg L, Pouillart P, Weiner R, Amiel JL, Hayat M, Jasmin C, De Wassal F (1974) Nonspecific immune responses in hematosarcomas and acute leukemias. In: Mathe G, Weiner R (eds) Investigations and stimulation of immunity of cancer patients. Springer, Berlin Heidelberg New York, pp 42-53 (Recent Results in Cancer Research, vol 47)

558. Schnitzer B, Kass L (1973) Leukemia phase of reticulum cell sarcoma (histiocytic lymphoma). A clinicopathologic and ultrastructural study. Cancer 31: 547-559

559. Schouten JL, Weese JL, Carbone PP (1981) Lymphoma of the breast. Ann Surg 6: 749-753

560. Schreiber G, Habighorst LV, Albers P, Eilers H (1977) Lymphogranulomatose des Esophagus. Fortschr Röntgenstr 126: 495-496

561. Schwerk W, Braun B, Boger A, Schmitz-Moormann P (1977) Primares Hodgkin-Sarkom des Dünndarms bei Sprue-Syndrom mit Steatorrhoe. Z Gastroenterol 15: 240-245

562. Scully RE, Mark EJ, McNeely BU (1982) Case records of the Massachusetts General Hospital, no 47. N Engl J Med 307: 1391-1397

563. Seligman BR, Rosner F, Davenport J (1974) Primary lymphosarcoma of the parotid gland. Cancer 33: 239-243

564. Selke AC Jr, Jona JZ, Belin RP (1976) Massive enlargement of the ileocecal valve due to lymphoid hyperplasia. Am J Roentgenol 127: 518-520

565. Seltzer RA, Wenlund DE (1967) Renal lymphoma: arteriographic studies. Am J Roentgenol 101: 692-695

566. Seo IS, Kinkley WB, Warner TFCS, Warfel KA (1982) Combined morphologic and immunologic approach to the diagnosis of gastrointestinal lymphomas. I. Malignant lymphoma of the stomach (a clinicopathologic study of 22 cases). Cancer 49: 493-501

567. Severini A, Bellomi M, Cozzi G, Pizzetti P, Spinelli P (1981) Lymphomatous involvement of intrahepatic and extrahepatic biliary ducts. PTC

and ERCP findings. Acta Radiol [Diagn] 22: 159-163

568. Shands WC, Gatling RR (1970) Cancer of the thyroid: review of 109 cases. Ann Surg 171: 735-745

569. Shani A, Schutt AJ, Weiland LH (1978) Primary gastric malignant lymphoma followed by gastric adenocarcinoma. Report of 4 cases and review of the literature. Cancer 42: 2039-2044

570. Sherrick DW, Hodgson JR, Dockerty MB (1965) The roentgenologic diagnosis of primary gastric lymphoma. Radiology 84: 925-932

571. Shimkin PM, Sagerman RH (1969) Lymphoma of the thyroid gland. Radiology 92: 812-816

572. Shin KH, Lott JS, Corbett WE, Garret PG (1976) Malignant lymphoma of the thyroid gland. Can J Surg 19: 442-445

573. Shiraki T, Kinoshita S, Kawasaki H, Miyaoka T, Tanizawa Y, Toriyama T, Kuroiwa N, Kubota O, Tada M, Akasaka Y (1975) Two cases of primary malignant lymphoma of the large bowel. Jpn J Gastroenterol 75: 1404-1410

574. Shirkhoda A, Staab EV, Mittelstaedt CA (1980) Renal lymphoma imaged by ultrasound and Gallium 67. Radiology 137: 175-180

575. Shukla HS, Misra MC (1979) Dysphagia in Hodgkin's disease. A case report. Clin Oncol 5: 371-381

576. Shuman LS, Libshitz HI (1984) Solid pleural manifestations of lymphoma. Am J Roentgenol 142: 269-273

577. Sichez JP, Raphael M, Leporrier M, Kujas M, Nguyen JP, Vaneffenterre R, Nachanakian A (1982) Compressions médullaires tumorales dans les hémopathies malignes. Ann Med Int 133: 251-255

578. Siekavizza JL, Bernardino ME, Samaan NA (1981) Suprarenal mass and its differential diagnosis. Urology 18: 625-632

579. Silber SJ, Chang CY (1973) Primary lymphoma of kidney. J Urol 110: 282-284

580. Siler J, Hunter TB, Weiss J, Haber K (1980) Increased echogenicity of the spleen in benign and malignant disease. Am J Roentgenol 134: 1011-1014

581. Silvis SE, Rohrmann CA, Vennes JA (1976) Diagnostic accuracy of endoscopic retrograde cholangiopancreatography in hepatic, biliary and pancreatic malignancy. Ann Intern Med 84: 438-440

582. Simon G (1967) Intrathoracic Hodgkin's disease. Part 1: less common intra-thoracic manifestations of Hodgkin's disease. Br J Radiol 40: 926-929

583. Simonpietri JP (1978) Les localisations osseuses révélatrices de la maladie de Hodgkin. A propos de trois observations. Thesis Paris, Val de Marne

584. Singh A, Strobos RJ, Singh BM, Rothballer AB, Reddy V, Puljic S, Poon TP (1982) Steroid-induced remissions in CNS lymphoma. Neurology 32: 1267-1271

585. Smith J, O'Connel RS, Huvos AG, Woodward HQ (1980) Hodgkin's disease complicated by radiation sarcoma in bone. Br J Radiol 53: 314-321

586. Snoddy WT (1952) Primary lymphosarcoma of the stomach. Gastroenterology 20: 537-553

587. Sondag D, Baumann R, Lacroute J, Schutz JF, Bergerat JP, Weill-Bousson M, Weill JP (1982) Lymphomes malins non hodgkiniens primitifs de l'estomac. A propos de 18 cas. Intérêt de la fibroscopie et discussion de l'attitude thérapeutique. Ann Gastroenterol Hepatol 18: 115-123

588. Spagnoli I, Gattoni F, Viganotti G (1982) Roentgenographic aspects of non-Hodgkin's lymphomas presenting with osseous lesions. Skeletal Radiol 8: 39-41

589. Spagnoli I, Viganotti G, Uslenghi C (1981) Le lymphome malin primitif de la vessie. A propos d'un cas. Ann Radiol 24: 219-220

590. Spence WJE, Ritchie S (1969) Lymphomas of small bowel and their relationship to idiopathic steatorrhea. Can J Surg 12: 207-209

591. Spillane JA, Kendall BE, Moseley IF (1982) Cerebral lymphoma: clinical-radiological correlation. J Neurol Neurosurg Psychiatry 45: 199-208

592. Stark P (1981) Bronchoenteric fistulae in lymphoma. Am J Roentgenol 136: 615-617

593. Steiner RM, Harell GS, Glatstein E, Wexler L (1970) Repeat lymphangiography in Hodgkin's disease. Radiology 97: 613-618

594. Stewart JR, Fajardo LF (1971) Radiation induced heart disease. Clinical and experimental aspects. Radiol Clin North Am 9: 511-531

595. Stolberg HO, Patt NL, Mac Ewen KF, Warwick TC (1964) Hodgkin's disease of the lung. Roentgenologic-pathologic correlation. Am J Roentgenol 92: 96-115

596. Strauss DJ, Filippa DA, Liebermann PH, Koziner B, Thaler T, Clarkson BD (1983) The non-Hodgkin's lymphomas. I. A retrospective clinical and pathological analysis of 499 cases diagnosed between 1958 and 1969. Cancer 51: 101-109

597. Strauss J, Magnet JL, Guerrin J, Fargeot P (1978) Les localisations osseuses de la maladie de Hodgkin et des lymphomes malins. Rhumatologie 30: 115-121

598. Strickland B (1967) Intrathoracic Hodgkin's disease. Part II. Peripheral manifestations of Hodgkin's disease in the chest. Br J Radiol 40: 930-938

599. Sufrin G, Keogh B, Moore RH, Murphy GP (1977) Secondary involvement of the bladder in malignant lymphoma. J Urol 118: 251-253

600. Sutton TJ, Gauthier N, Hassan M (1975) Les localisations rénales des lymphosarcomes de l'enfant. J Radiol 56: 685-690

601. Tadmor R, Davis KR, Roberson GH, Kleinman GM (1978) CT in primary malignant lymphoma

of the brain. J Comput Assist Tomogr 2: 135-140

602. Taleb N, Khouri K, Nassar W (1975) Les lymphomes à localisation digestive primitive. Considérations cliniques, radiologiques et thérapeutiques à propos de 42 observations. J Med Liban 28: 233-258

603. Talvalkar GV (1973) Primary lymphosarcoma of the breast: a report of 10 cases. Indian J Cancer 10: 322-329

604. Taylor I (1976) Malignant lymphoma of the thyroid. Br J Surg 63: 932-933

605. Teillet F, Boiron M, Bernard J (1971) A reappraisal of clinical and biological signs in staging of Hodgkin's disease. Cancer Res 31: 1723-1729

606. Tepperman BS, Gospodarowicz MK, Bush RS, Brown TC (1982) Non-Hodgkin lymphoma of the testis. Radiology 142: 203-208

607. Terz JJ, Farr HW (1969) Primary lymphosarcoma of the tonsil. Surgery 65: 772-776

608. The Non-Hodgkin's Lymphoma Pathologic Classification Project (1982) National Cancer Institute sponsored study of classifications of non-Hodgkin's lymphomas. Summary and description of a working formulation for clinical usage. Cancer 49: 2112-2135

609. Thomas JL, Bernardino ME, Vermess M, Barnes PA, Fuller LM, Hagemeister FB, Doppman J, Fisher RI, Longo DL (1982) EOE-13 in the detection of hepatosplenic lymphoma. Radiology 145: 629-634

610. Thomas M, MacPherson P (1982) CT of intracranial lymphoma. Clin Radiol 33: 331-336

611. Thorbjarnarson B, Beal JM, Pearce JM (1956) Primary malignant lymphoid tumors of the stomach. Cancer 9: 712-717

612. Ti M, Elquezabal A, Dosik H (1975) Lymphosarcoma of the breast. Am J Med Sci 269: 409-413

613. Tori G (1951) Osservazioni clinico statistiche e considerazioni critiche intorno alla radioterapia dei tumori rinofaringei. Radiol Radioter Fis Med 4: 121-136

614. Touboul E, Fauchon F, Gardeur D, Foncin JF, Philippon J, Merle-Beral H, Guerin RA (1983) Lymphome primitif du système nerveux central. Sem Hôp Paris 59: 365-371

615. Tracy GP, Brown DE, Johnson LW, Gottlieb AS (1974) Radiation-induced coronary artery disease. JAMA 228: 1660-1662

616. Travail Collectif Effectué dans le Cadre de la Société de Gastroentérologie de l'Ouest (1982) Lymphomes malins primitifs non hodgkiniens du tube digestif. Ann Gastroenterol Hepatol 18: 97-113

617. Tristant H, Laval-Jeantet M, Katz M, Dumont J, Dufillot C, Chelloul N (1974) Apports séméiologiques de la lymphographie pédieuse dans les sarcomes ganglionnaires. J Radiol 55: 199-203

618. Tristant H, Laval-Jeantet M, Katz M, Weisgerber C, Teillet F (1975) Localisations de la maladie de Hodgkin à la coupole diaphragmatique. Ann Radiol 18: 641-648

619. Trokel SL, Hilal SK (1980) Submillimeter resolution in CT scan of orbital disease. Ophthalmology 87: 412-417

620. Trotman BW, Glick JH, Debarros SGS, Atkinson BF (1980) Dysphagia in a patient with Hodgkin's disease. JAMA 244: 2552-2553

621. Trump DL, Mann RB (1982) Diffuse large cell and undifferentiated lymphomas with prominent mediastinal involvement. A poor prognostic subset of patients with non-Hodgkin's lymphoma. Cancer 50: 277-282

622. Tschang TP (1976) Nodular malignant lymphoma and amyloidosis. A case report. Cancer 38: 2192-2196

623. Turner RR, Colby TV, Mackintosh FR (1981) Testicular lymphomas: a clinicopathologic study of 35 cases. Cancer 48: 2095-2102

624. Twiford TX, Zornoza J, Libshitz HI (1978) Recurrent spontaneous pneumothorax after radiation therapy to the thorax. Chest 73: 387-388

625. Tylen U (1975) Angiography in disease of the peripancreatic lymph nodes. Acta Radiol [Diagn] 16: 625-632

626. Vadrot D, Laval-Jeantet M, Vadrot M, Delmas PF, Bouzac H (1978) L'échotomographie dans l'étude des adénopathies abdominales. Techniques d'examen et séméiologie. J Radiol 59: 399-406

627. Valavanis A, Friedel R, Schubiger O, Hayek J (1979) Cerebral granulomatous angiitis simulating brain tumor. J Comput Assist Tomogr 3: 436-538

628. Van Den Heule B, Taylor CR, Terry R, Lukes RJ (1982) Présentation of malignant lymphoma in the rectum. Cancer 49: 2602-2607

629. Vanel D, Bayle C, Hartmann O, Rebibo G, Tamman S (1982) Radiological study of two disseminated malignant non-Hodgkin lymphomas affecting only the bones in children. Skeletal Radiol 9: 83-87

630. Vanel D, Couanet D, Piekarski JD, Masselot J (1983) Radiological findings in 23 pediatric cases of malignant histiocytosis. Eur J Radiol 3: 60-62

631. Van Slyck EJ, Schuman BM (1972) Lymphocytic lymphosarcoma of the gallbladder. Cancer 30: 810-816

632. Van Regemorter G (1973) Obstruction de l'uretère lombo-iliaque: première manifestation des cancers non urinaires. J Urol Nephrol 79: 262-266

633. Vasquez Quevedo F, Val Bernal F, Perez de la Lastra L, Garijo F, Castanedo M, Castillo J, Martinez Barona J (1980) Linfomas no Hodgkinianos, primitivos, de intestino delgado (revision de 12 casos). Rev Esp Enf Ap Digest 57: 133-148

634. Velentjas E, Barrett A, Mac Elwain TJ, Peckham MJ (1980) Mediastinal involvement in early-stage Hodgkin's disease. Response to treatment and pattern of relapse. Eur J Cancer 16: 1065-1068

635. Vermess M, Bernardino ME, Doppman JL, Fisher RI, Thomas JL, Velasquez WS, Fuller LM, Russo A (1981) Use of intravenous liposoluble contrast material for the examination of the liver and spleen in lymphoma. J Comput Assist Tomogr 5: 709-713

636. Vessal K, Dutz W, Kohout E, Rezvani L (1980) Immunoproliferative small intestinal disease with duodenojejunal lymphoma: radiologic changes. Am J Roentgenol 135: 491-497

637. Vieta JO, Friedl HL, Craver LF (1942) A survey of Hodgkin's disease and lymphosarcoma in bone. Radiology 39: 1-14

638. Viganotti G, Bergonzi S, Guzzon A, Coopmans de Yoldi G, Farina F (1982) Diagnostica radiologica e teletermografica dei linfomi mammari (28 casi). Radiol Med (Torino) 68: 455-462

639. Wagonfeld JB, Baker AL, Reed JS, Platz CE, Kirsner JB (1976) Acute dilatation of the colon in malignant lymphoma. Gastroenterology 70: 264-267

640. Walker JH, Schulz MD (1947) Carcinoma of tonsil; review of treatment and its results in a group of ninety cases. Radiology 49: 162-167

641. Walt AJ, Woolner LB, Black BM (1957) Primary malignant lymphoma of the thyroid. Cancer 10: 663-677

642. Wang CC (1969) Malignant lymphoma of Waldeyer's ring. Radiology 92: 1335-1339

643. Wang CC (1971) Primary malignant lymphoma of the oral cavity and paranasal sinuses. Radiology 100: 151-153

644. Wang CC (1972) Malignant lymphoma of the larynx. Laryngoscope 82: 97-100

645. Wang CC, Petersen JA (1956) Malignant lymphoma of the gastroinestinal tract: roentgenographic consideration. Acta Radiol [Diagn] 46: 523-532

646. Wang CC, Scully RE, Leadbetter WF (1969) Primary malignant lymphoma of the urinary bladder. Cancer 24: 772-776

647. Weick JK, Kiely JM, Harrison EG, Carr DT, Scanlon PW (1973) Pleural effusion in lymphoma. Cancer 31: 848-853

648. Weimar G, Culp DA, Loening S, Narayana A (1981) Urogenital involvement by malignant lymphomas. J Urol 125: 230-231

649. Weissman IL, Warnker R, Butcher EC, Rouse R, Levy R (1978) The lymphoid system; its normal architecture and the potential for the understanding of the system through the study of lymphoproliferative disease. Hum Pathol 9: 25-45

650. Weyman PJ, Koehler RE (1980) Diffuse colonic nodularity and splenomegaly. Invest Radiol 15: 2-5

651. Whitaker D (1976) The role of cytology in the detection of malignant lymphoma of the uterine cervix. Acta Cytol 20: 510-513

652. White AA, Palubinskas AJ (1970) Renal Hodgkin's disease. Angiographic demonstration. Radiology 96: 551-552

653. Wig JD, Kohli PK, Kaushik SP, Talwar BL, Bushwarmath SR, Dutta TK (1980) Unusual cause of massive rectal bleeding. Indian J Cancer 17: 276-278

654. Williams RS, Crowell RM, Fisher M, Davis K, Lavyne MH, Ropper AH, Bremer AM (1979) Clinical and radiologic remission in reticulum cell sarcoma of the brain. Arch Neurol 36: 206-210

655. Williams SLH, Anastopulos HP, Presant CA (1969) Selective renal arteriography in Hodgkin's disease of the kidney. A case report. Radiology 93: 1059-1060

656. Winter CC, Puente E, Wall RL (1979) Bladder involvement with lymphoma. Urology 14: 151-153

657. Wintrobe MM (ed) (1981) Clinical hematology. Febiger, Philadelphia

658. Wiseman C, Liao KT (1972) Primary lymphoma of the breast. Cancer 29: 1705-1712

659. Witten DM, Myers GH Jr, Utz DC (1977) Emmett's clinical urography. Saunders, Philadelphia, pp 1541-1549

660. Wolfe JD, Trevor ED, Kjeldsberg CR (1980) Pulmonary manifestations of mycosis fungoïdes. Cancer 46: 2648-2653

661. Wong DS, Fuller LM, Butler JJ, Shullenberger CC (1975) Extranodal non-Hodgkin's lymphomas of the head and neck. Radiology 123: 471-481

662. Wood NL, Coltman CA (1973) Localized primary extranodal Hodgkin's disease. Ann Intern Med 78: 113-118

663. Woodruff JD, Noli Castillo RD, Novack ER (1963) Lymphoma of the ovary. A study of 35 cases from the ovarian tumor registry of the American Gynecological Society. Am J Obstet Gynecol 85: 912-918

664. Woolner LB, Mac Conahey WM, Beahrs OH, Marden Black B (1966) Primary malignant lymphoma of the thyroid. Review of forty-six cases. Am J Surg 111: 502-523

665. Worthy TS (1981) Evaluation of diagnostic laparotomy and splenectomy in Hodgkin's disease (report no 12). Clin Radiol 32: 523-526

666. Wright CJE (1973) Solitary malignant lymphoma of the uterus. Am J Obstet Gynecol 117: 114-120

667. Wychulis AR, Beahrs OH, Wollner LB (1966) Malignant lymphoma of the colon. A study of 69 cases. Arch Surg 93: 215-225

668. Wyman SM, Weber AL (1969) Calcification in intrathoracic nodes in Hodgkin's disease. Radiology 93: 1021-1024

669. Yahalom J, Hasin Y, Fuks Z (1983) Acute myocardial infarction with normal coronary arteriogram after mantle field radiation therapy for Hodgkin's disease. Cancer 52: 637–641
670. Yeh S (1962) A historical classification of carcinoma of the nasopharynx with a critical review as to the existence of the lymphoepitheliomas. Cancer 15: 895–920
671. Yeo JH, Jakobiec FA, Abbott GF, Trokel SL (1982) Combined clinical and computed tomographic diagnosis of orbital lymphoid tumors. Am J Ophthalmol 94: 235–245
672. Young IF, Roberts-Thomson IC, Sullivan JR (1981) Histiocytic lymphoma presenting with extrahepatic biliary obstruction: a report of three cases. Aust NZ J Surg 51: 181–183
673. Young RC, Canellos GP, Chabner BA, Hubbard SM, DeVita V (1978) Patterns of relapse in advanced Hodgkin's disease: treatment with combination radiotherapy. Cancer 42: 1001–1007
674. Zeller C, Schmutz G, Giron JP, Kempf F (1983) Aspects radiologiques des localisations rectales et coliques des lymphomes non hodgkiniens. A propos de 30 cas. J Radiol 64: 233–239
675. Zeller C, Schmutz G, Pauline D, Giron JP, Kempf F (1983) Aspects radiologiques des localisations gastriques des lymphomes malins non hodgkiniens. A propos de 50 observations. J Radiol 64: 225–232
676. Zenny JC, Aim D, Grenier P, Bernard JF, Nahum H (1980) Les localisations sternales de la maladie de Hodgkin. A propos de deux cas. J Radiol 61: 281–283
677. Ziegler JL (1981) Burkitt's lymphoma. N Engl J Med 305: 735–745
678. Zimmerman LE (1964) Lymphoid tumors. In: Toniuk M (ed) Ocular and adnexal tumors: new and controversial aspects. Mosby, Saint Louis, pp 429–446
679. Zornoza J, Dodd GD (1980) Lymphoma of the gastrointestinal tract. Sem Roentgenol 15: 272–287
680. Zornoza J, Ginaldi S (1981) Computed tomography in hepatic lymphoma. Radiology 138: 405–410
681. Zornoza J, Cabanillas FF, Altoff TM, Ordonez N, Cohen MA (1981) Percutaneous needle biopsy in abdominal lymphoma. Am J Roentgenol 136: 97–103